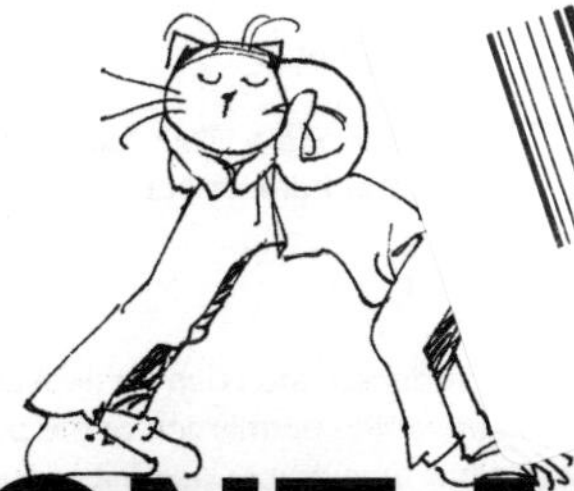

THE ONE MINUTE EXERCISE BOOK

NO GYM, NO LEOTARD, NO SWEAT!

Toni Goffe

Hodder & Stoughton
LONDON SYDNEY AUCKLAND

First published in Great Britain in 2005

10 9 8 7 6 5 4 3 2 1

British Library Cataloguing in Publication Data
A record for this book is available from the British Library

ISBN 0 340 86402 8

Printed and bound in Great Britain by CPI Bath

The paper and board used in this paperback are natural recyclable products made from wood grown in sustainable forests. The manufacturing processes conform to the environmental regulations of the country of origin.

Hodder & Stoughton
A Division of Hodder Headline Ltd
338 Euston Road
London NW1 3BH
www.madaboutbooks.com

CONTENTS

ACKNOWLEDGEMENTS

I'd like to thank Jenny Gove, Tim Laskey and Sue Woodd for their help with this book.

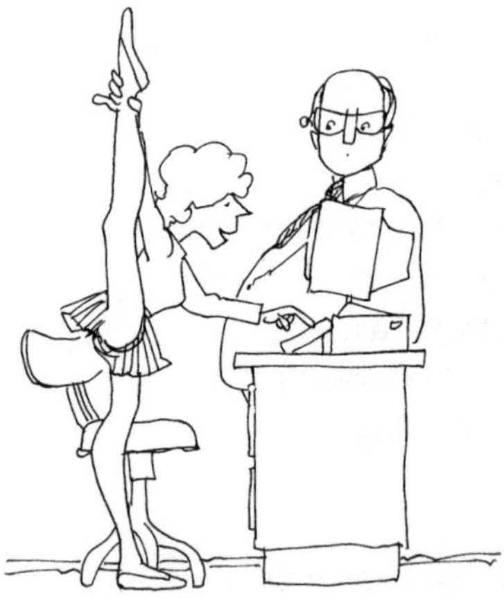

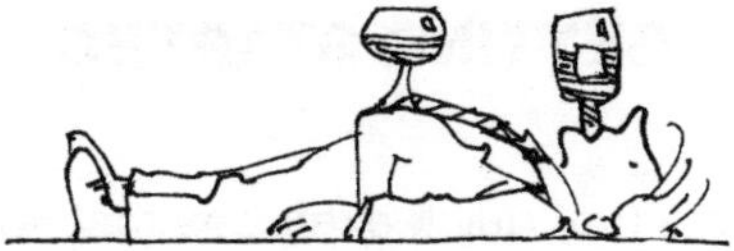

INTRODUCTION

Everyone knows that exercise is good for you but who has the time to do any? The working day seems to be getting longer and busier, and when you finally drag yourself home after a hard day's work, exercise is the last thing you want to think about. More likely, a stiff drink and a lie-down.

Do you remember the coming of the computer to the workplace? It was supposed to halve the working day and give us more leisure time to spend on healthy exercise and having fun. Well, we all know that the reverse is the truth.

So, how can we find any time to exercise? With the help of this book, of course!

GETTING STARTED

I have devised a system of quick exercises that you can do anywhere and at any spare moment you have. They only last a minute at a time so you don't have to spend any time worrying about what to wear, which gym to go to, etc., etc. You can just do them where you are!

You might be surprised to find out how many spare moments there are in a working day, when you are waiting for something to happen. Moments such as waiting for your turn in the queue for the loo, or waiting for your computer to download, waiting for a bus, a train or a plane, or waiting for your boss to stop talking to you so you can get on with some work. All moments when you could be doing one of your *one-minute exercises*!

Let's get on with the first exercises ...

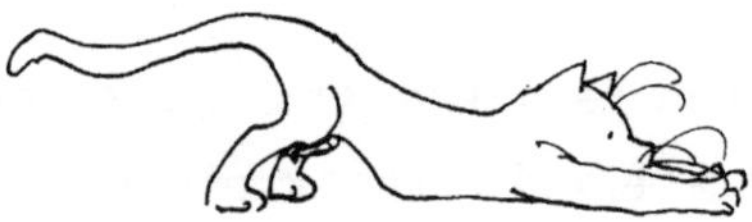

EXERCISES YOU CAN DO IN BED

When your alarm goes off in the morning is there a moment of indecision? 'Shall I get up?' or 'Shall I just lie here?' or 'Shall I hurl the alarm clock across the room and go back to sleep?' Then you start to think about the day ahead. 'Shall I call in sick?' and so on, and by the time you do get up you feel awful and negative, not at all ready to face the day ahead.

If this happens to you every morning then try this. Start your day with *exercises you can do in bed*! They will take your mind off work and get your mind and body ready to feel more positive and energised. And you don't even have to get up yet!

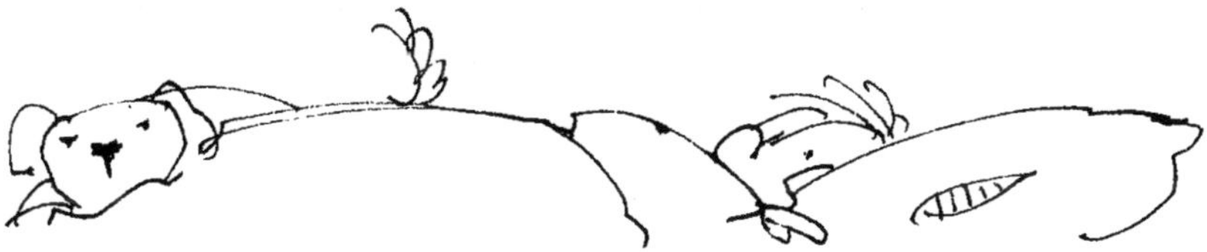

Breathing

Let's start with *breathing*. You are probably doing this naturally but the breathing I'm talking about is *deep breathing*.

Lie on your back and place your hands on your stomach. Breathe through your nose and relax all your muscles. Now when you breathe in, let your stomach expand before filling the lungs with air. Then let the air out gently. You can try counting to ten. This may be difficult at first so try a count of five in and five out. Later, when you get used to this way of breathing, you can extend the time. So, if you get to a count of ten, repeat it five times, or if it's five, then eleven times, making the time up to a *one-minute exercise*!

Now you've completed your first minute exercise of the day, are you ready to go to the second minute of your exercise programme?

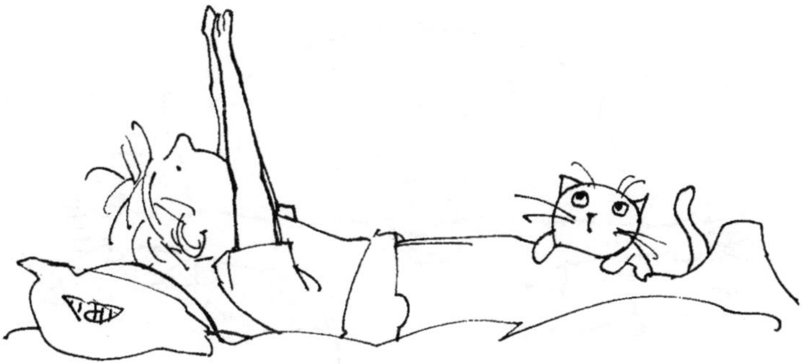

Stretching

Still lying on your back, stretch your arms out in front of you at shoulder level and push towards the ceiling, hollowing your back. Try to reach the ceiling in your mind and then let your shoulders return to the bed and relax. Count to ten up and relax for ten. Repeat twice.

Time: One minute

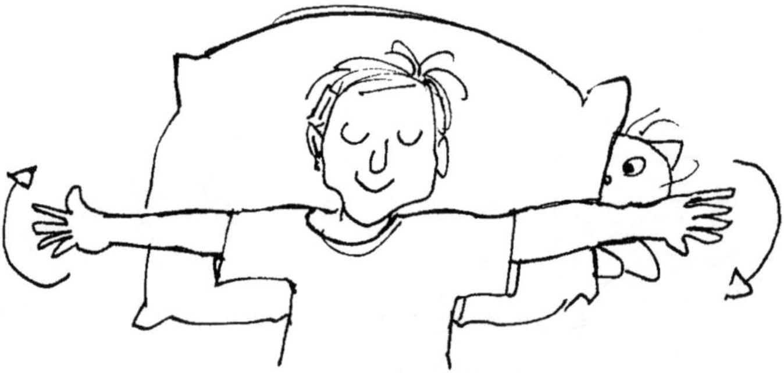

More Stretching

Stretch your arms to the side at shoulder height. Be careful not to strike a partner or pet or knock the alarm clock flying.

Push out as far as you can and count to ten. Now add a twist. Turn one hand, palm up, as far as you can. While doing this, turn your other hand the other way, palm down, to get a good twist in your arms. Count to ten. Now reverse which way the arms are twisting. Repeat twice on each side.

Time: One minute

Even More Stretching

Shove yourself down in the bed so you can push your arms above your head and push your legs out as far as you can, heels first. Count to ten. Repeat twice.

To add to this exercise, stretch again, but this time push out one arm and the opposite leg. Now do the same with the opposite arm and leg. Count to ten. Repeat twice.

Time: One minute

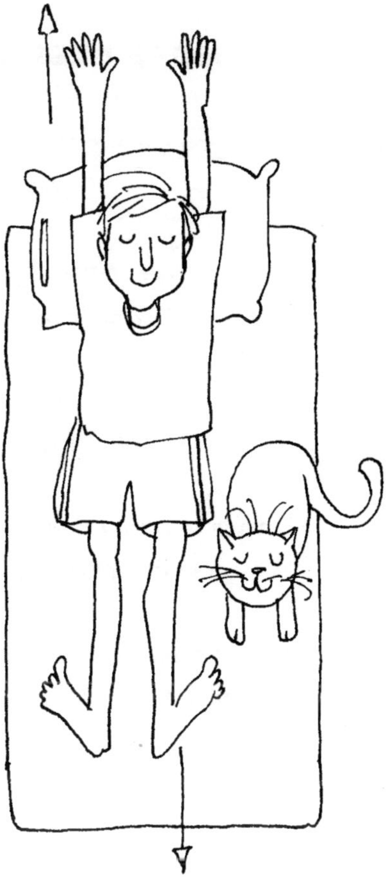

MORE EXERCISES YOU CAN DO IN BED

If you suffer from lower back pain, here are some exercises you can do before getting up.

Lie on your back, take a deep breath and relax. Bring one of your knees up to your chest and hold it there with both hands. Count to ten slowly. Now let the leg go and stretch it out. Bring the other knee up and repeat the exercise. Three on either side will give you your *one-minute work-out*.

This time bring up both legs and hold them to your chest. You can hold them there *for the full minute* to get a good stretch.

To add even more stretch, rotate your knees in a circular movement to the right ten times and then to the left ten times. Do this three times to give yourself a *one-minute exercise*.

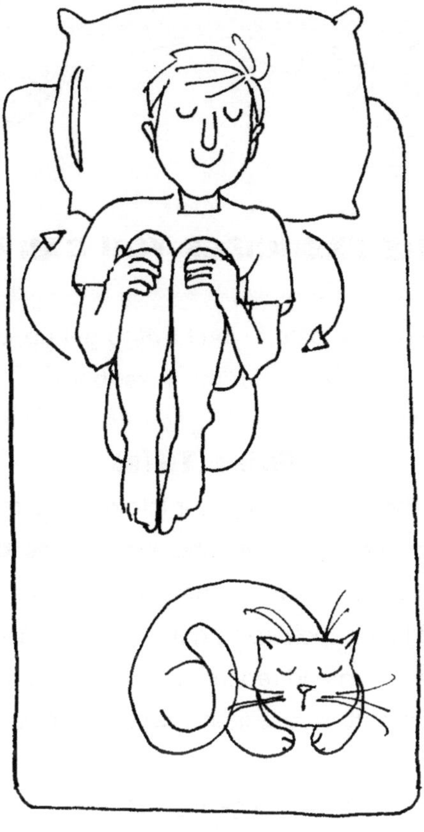

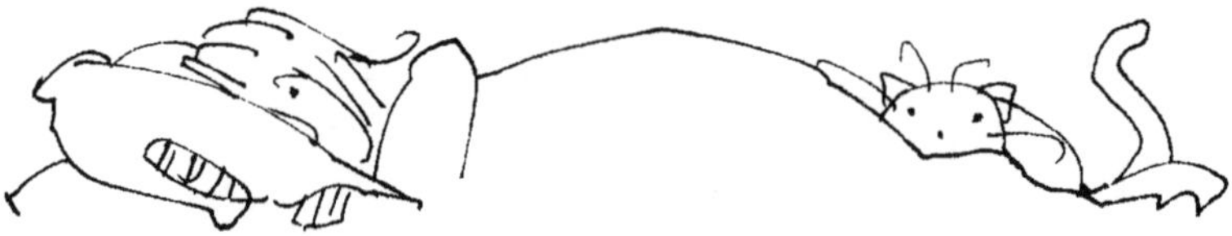

EVEN MORE EXERCISES YOU CAN DO IN BED

If you still have a minute before you have to get up, this is an excellent exercise for the lower back.

Spine Twist

Lie on your back and bring your left knee up to your chest, holding it there with your right hand. Now let the knee drop to the right and hold it gently down on the bed with your right hand. Keep your left shoulder on the bed to get a full diagonal stretch in your spine. Count to ten and repeat on the other side. Three times on both side will only take *one minute*!

Now, it's getting-up time!

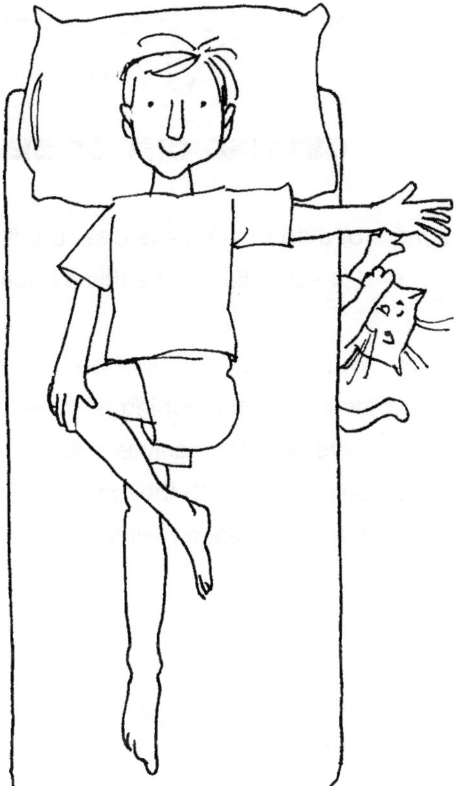

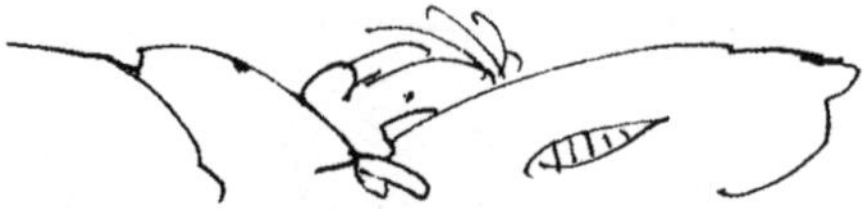

GETTING OUT OF BED

This is more of a tip than an exercise, but it would be good if you could make this a habit.

There are many ways of getting out of bed. Some people just keep rolling till they fall to the floor, hoping that the shock of the fall will wake them up. Others drag themselves out, holding on to the nearest bedpost or door. Some push with their arms till they reach the bottom of the bed and then ease their way into their slippers.

Try this: Roll on to your side, facing the outside of your bed. By putting your legs in the air, swing them down and off the bed so you can sit up with your feet on the floor. Sit up straight and see if you can stand up *without* using your arms to help you. This is a good exercise for both your legs and your posture.

Think of pushing your feet into the floor to give you the lift you need to get on to your feet. Try adopting this when getting up from any chair. It's a good habit to get into.

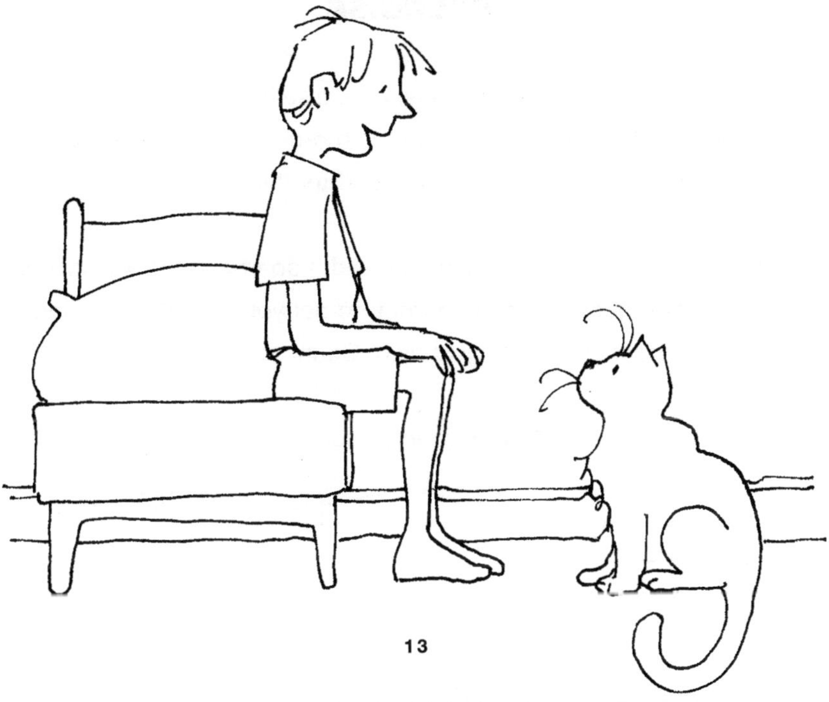

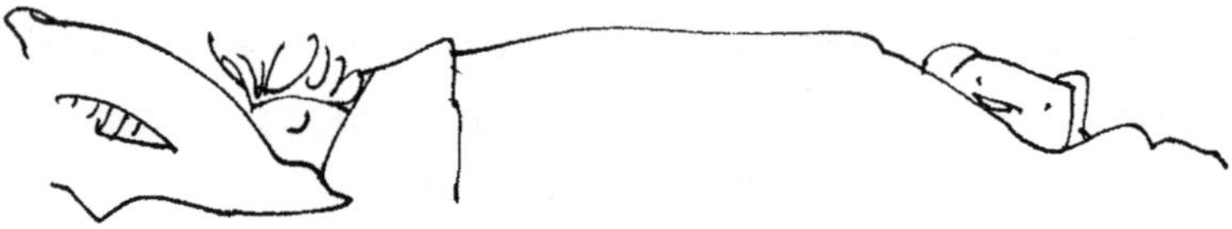

THE HOW-TO-WAKE-UP-IN-THE-MORNING EXERCISE

If you are like almost everyone else in this world, you have trouble waking up in the morning. Once you drag yourself out of the bed try this …

Stand with your legs about shoulder width apart and vigorously rub your hands together, back and front, to get your blood circulating. Massage your fingers also. Count to ten twice.

Time: Twenty seconds

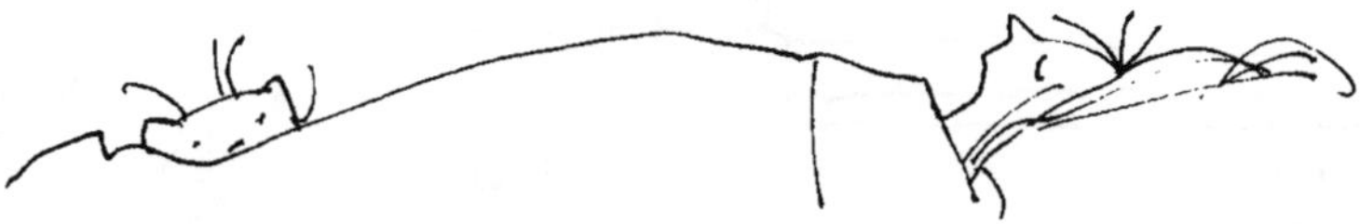

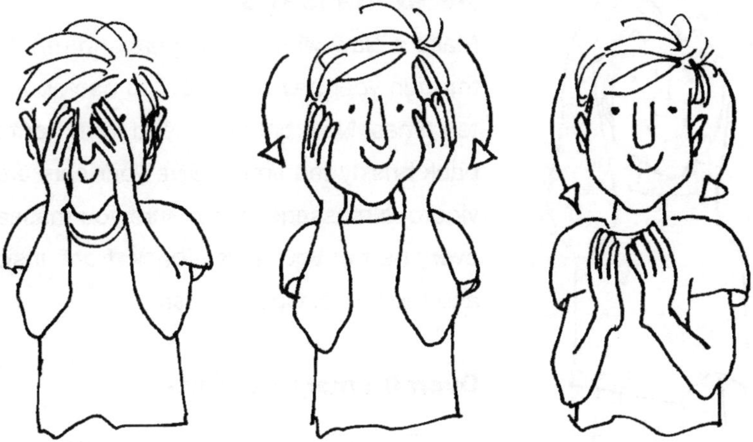

Face Massage

Now place your middle fingers on either side of your nose. Push up to the top of your forehead. With your hands covering your face, pull your hands down either side of your face to your chin. Repeat this movement nine times as quickly and briskly as you want to.

Time: Ten seconds

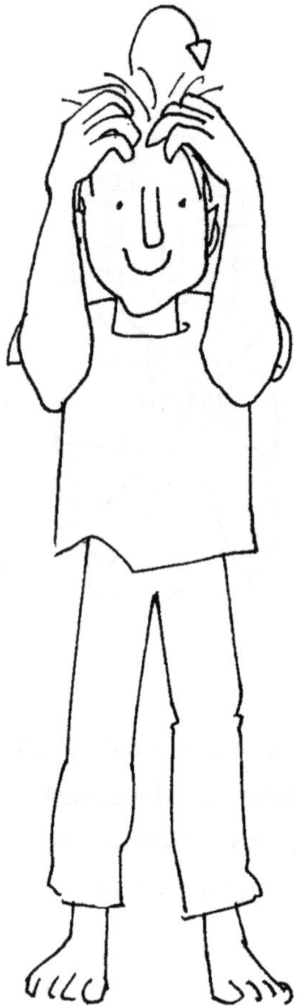

Head Massage

Make a claw with your fingers and run them through your hair from front to back briskly ten times. Now pat your head from front to back briskly ten times. Give your ears a fast, vigorous massage. Make sure you massage every part of your ears – back, front, insides and the lobes. Count to ten.

Overall time: One minute

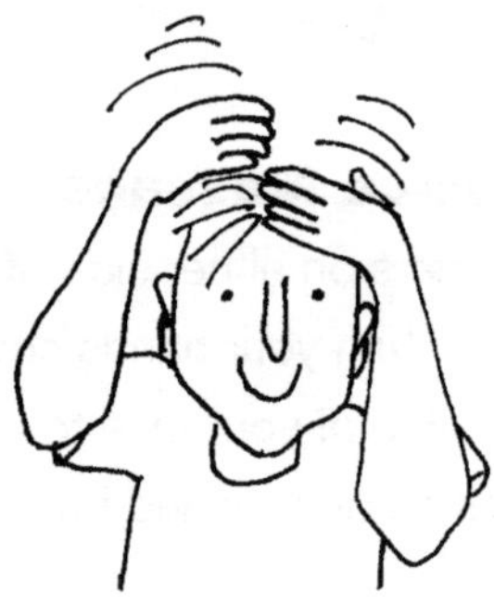

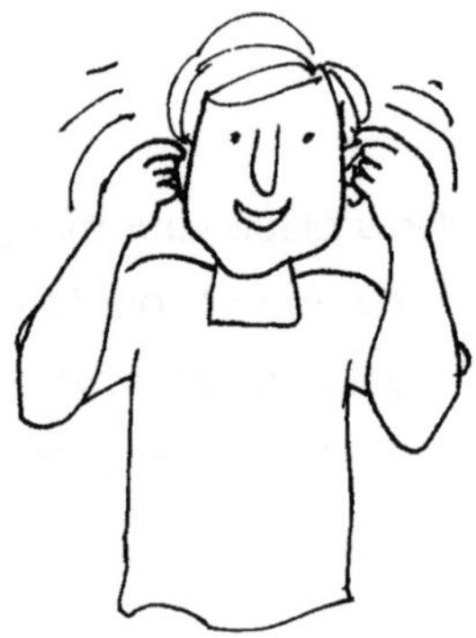

Now, if you *really* want to wake yourself up, add this to your programme…

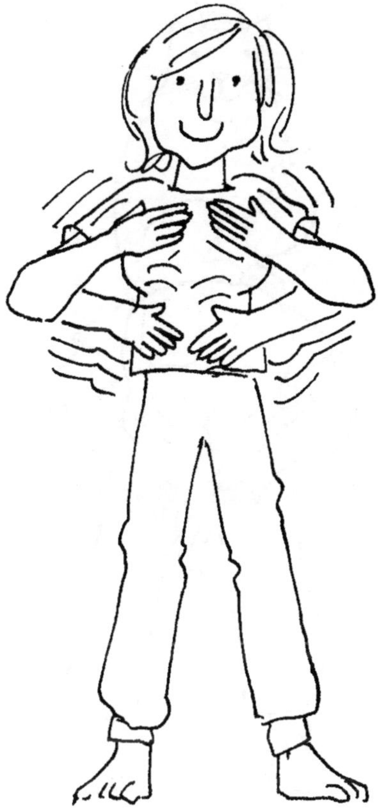

Slapping

Start with one hand slapping the back of your shoulder. The harder you can bear this, the better you will feel.

Bring your slapping hand to the front and top of your chest. Slap as much of the chest as you can with one hand, then change hands and do the other side. Return to the first side and slap down the back of your arms and up the insides. Do the other side. Repeat three times on each arm.

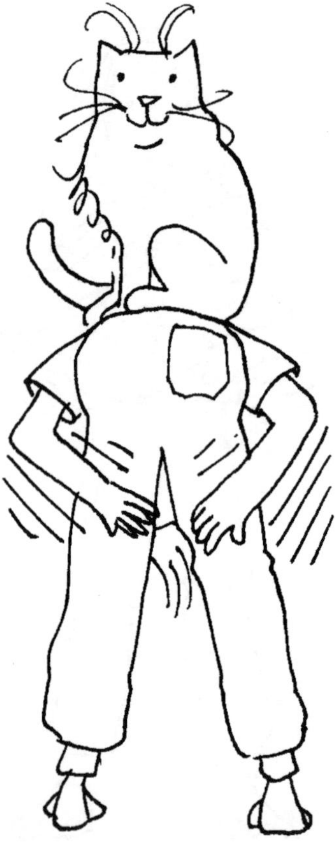

Now go back to your chest, down to the stomach, around to your buttocks and down the outsides of your legs, still slapping vigorously, and up the insides. Repeat three times.

This is quite a work-out and may well go over the prescribed minute. Think of it as an added extra, well worth the effort. You will feel fantastically refreshed afterwards. I guarantee it.

You may well want a rest after that tingling experience but if you want to complete the sequence add these exercises.

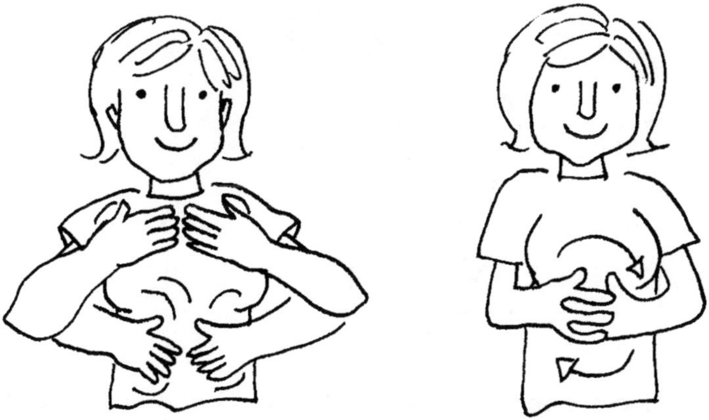

Massage

Massage your chest down to the stomach. Interlock your fingers and massage your stomach in a circular motion both clockwise and anti-clockwise. Repeat five times. Count to five in each direction.

Time: One minute

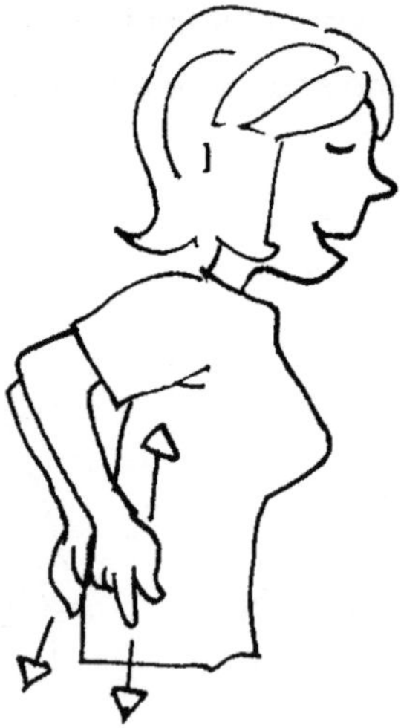

Give your kidneys a good rubbing with the backs of your hands. Bend your knees as you do this and bounce. Count to thirty.

Now move to the lower back and, using the backs of your thumbs, massage up and down your lower back. Count to thirty.

Time: One minute

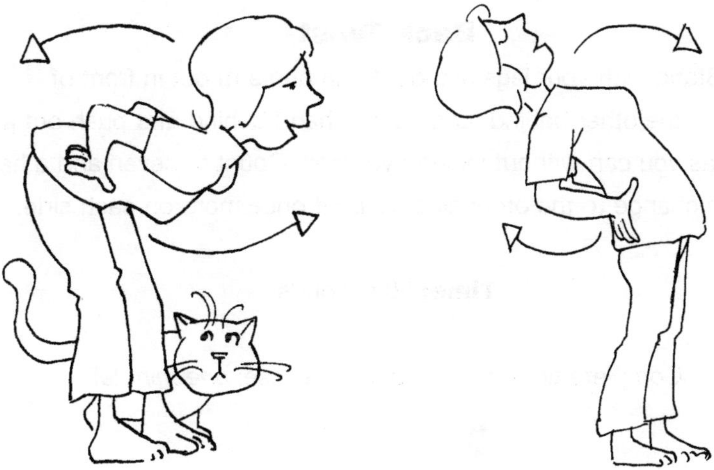

Back Work-Out

Put your hands on your hips and bend forward.
Bend your knees and bring your hips forward as you lean backwards, head up looking at the ceiling as your hips return to the upright position, giving your back a good S-shaped work-out.
Count to five each time and repeat five times.

Time: 30 seconds

Back Twist

Stand with your legs astride. Push one arm out in front of you and the other behind. Look at the hand behind and push out as much as you can without injuring yourself. Count to seven and a half then change to the other side. Repeat once more on each side.

Time: 30 seconds

Complete time for your back exercise: *one minute*!

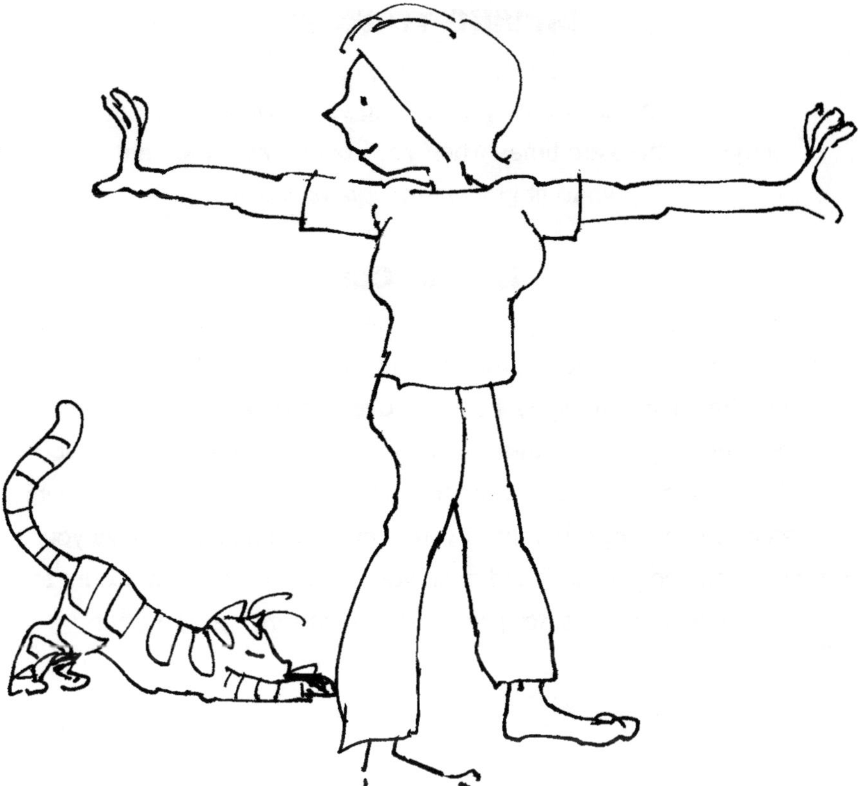

DRIVING TO WORK

Whenever you may be driving to the workplace, I'm sure there are times when you could grab a moment or two to fit in a *one-minute exercise*!

In Your Car

The part of your body that gets the least amount of exercise when driving a car is your legs. Although you seem to be using them all the time, they hang strangely, hovering over the pedals in limbo – not straight and not bent – with a lot of strain on the lower back. But you'll feel it in your legs first. So, when the next hold-up in the traffic occurs, stretch out your legs in front of you – remembering not to have your foot on the accelerator – and push your back into the seat. Count to five, twelve times, to give yourself a *one-minute exercise*!

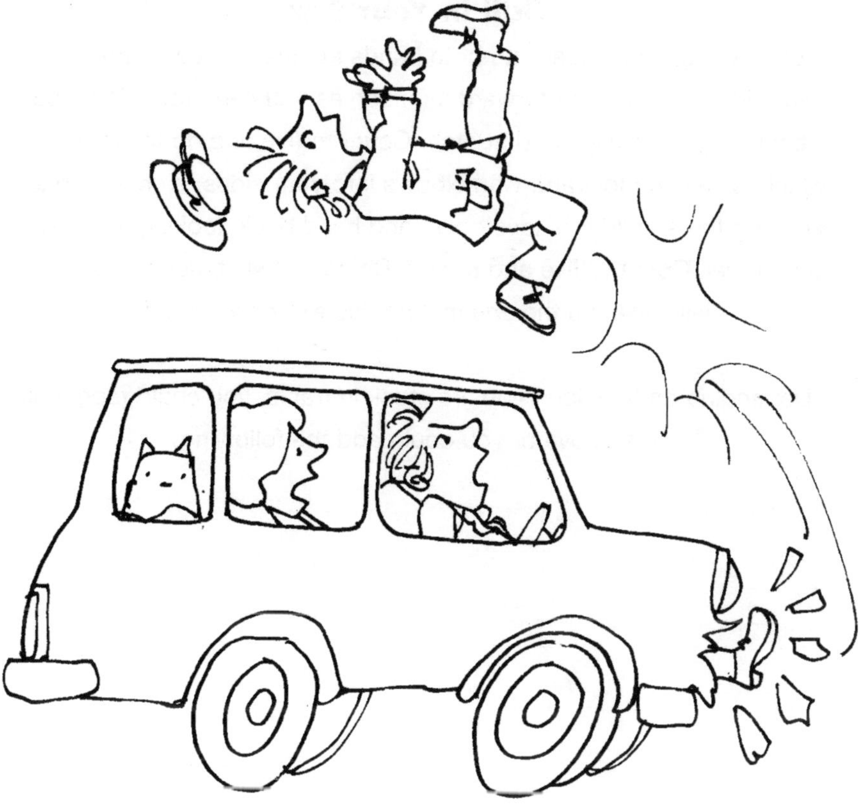

Still in Your Car

Hold the steering wheel with both hands at nine and three, and thrust your lower pelvis area forward as much as you can, 'rounding' your back to get a really good stretch. Count to five and do the reverse, which is: leaning forward, with elbows into your sides, arch your back, keeping the shoulder blades down and head back, looking at the roof of your car. Count to five and repeat. Doing this six times for each part will give you the *one minute* this exercise requires.

Depending on how long you are stuck in traffic, you could repeat all the above or you could add the following.

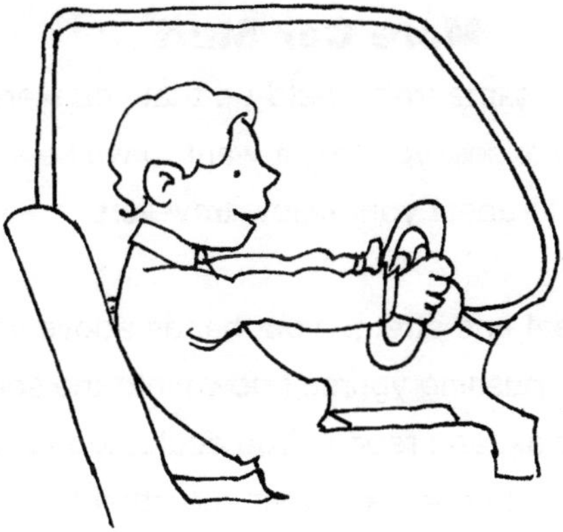

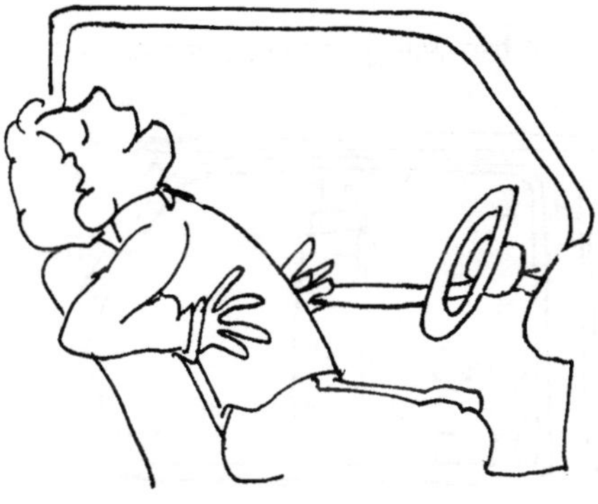

More Car Stuff

If you are in the same traffic hold-up that you were in doing the previous exercises, you might want to wait a while so not to upset your fellow travellers.

Sit up in your car seat and stretch your hands above your head. Push against the car roof, pushing yourself down into the seat. Hold for the count of ten; then relax, and repeat. You could add to this exercise by pushing more with one hand than the other to get a good side stretch, tipping your hip as you press.

Six counts of ten will give you the desired *one minute*.

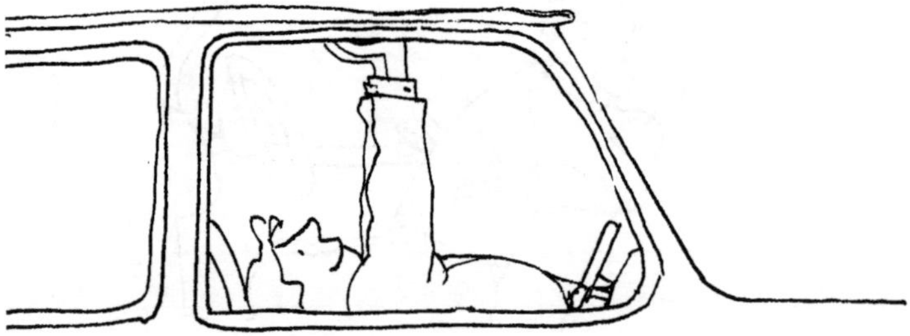

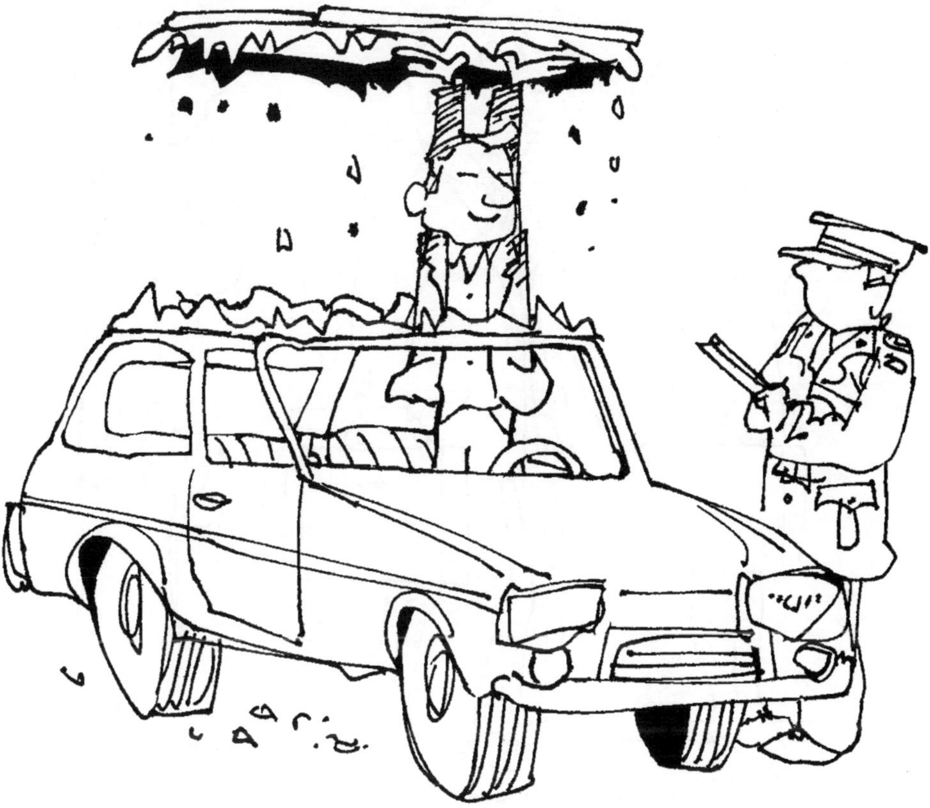

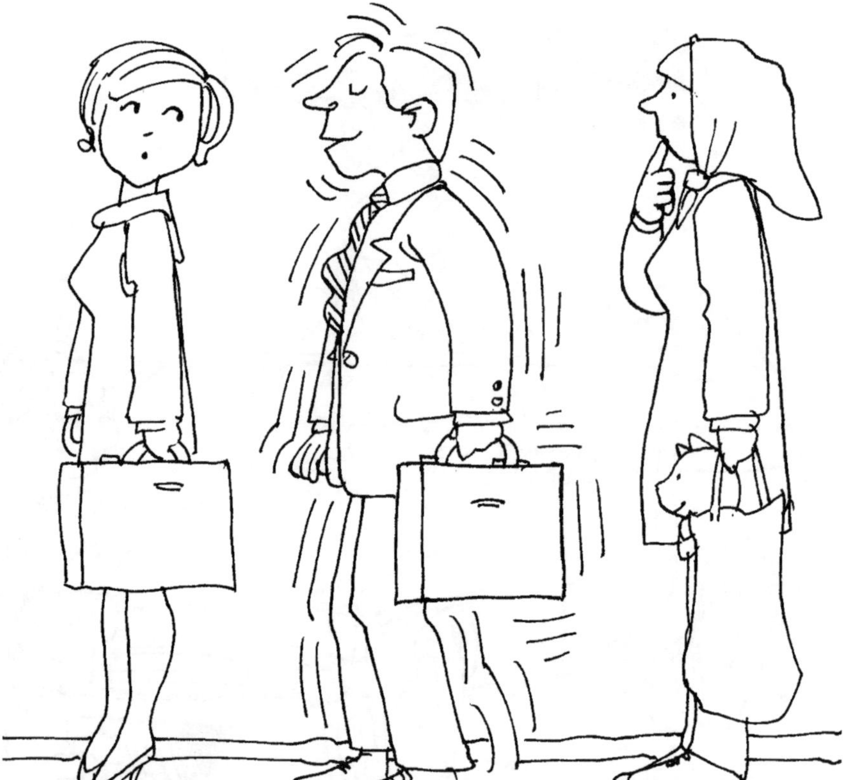

IN THE TRAIN OR BUS QUEUE

When you are in a queue for your train, bus or newspaper, try:

Bouncing

You just flex your knees and start a quickish up and down movement. This is to loosen up your joints so, as you bounce, check that your ankle joints are open and loose. When you are sure about them being loose, open and relaxed, move on to your knee joints. Check them out and then move on to your hips. Then your back, shoulders, neck, head and arms. Count one up and down movement as one second. Allow half a minute for a short queue, such as for a newspaper, but work this up to a minute at a time when finally you are in your train or bus and having to stand. If you get a seat, forget this exercise and have a good rest.

There is always a lot of waiting time when it comes to travelling by bus. A great opportunity for exercising. I am assuming that you will be carrying a briefcase or something similar. Be mindful of your fellow travellers.

The Briefcase Back Exercise

Stand in the queue with your legs astride, holding your briefcase in one hand. Let the weight of the briefcase pull you sideways, giving your opposite side a good stretch.

Take the hand holding your case down to your knee. Count to five. Change hands and try it again on the other side. Six times on either side will give you one minute, if your fellow travellers will let you. If there is a bad reaction, stop. If not, go on to the next extension.

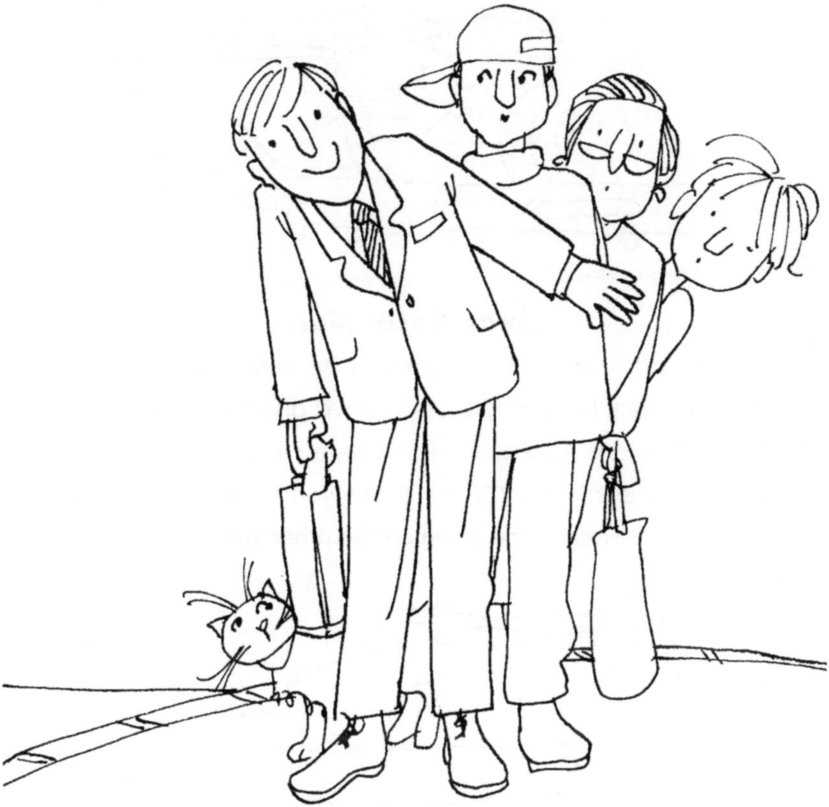

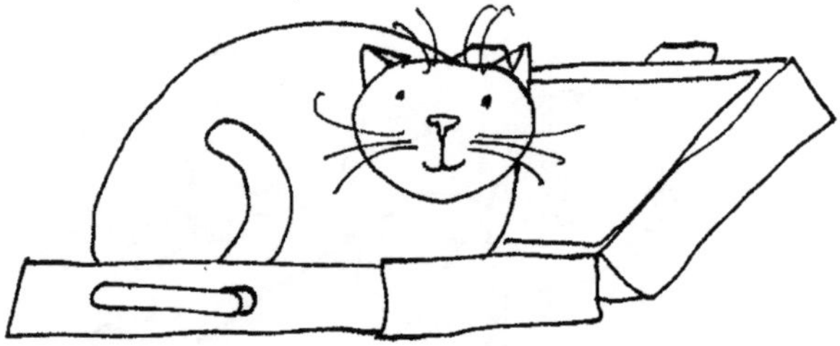

Back Extension

This time, hold the briefcase over the side of your head and let your back bend sideways. This will give you an even greater stretch than before. As you count to five, try to get more stretch into your back to every count. Ten will give you a really good stretch. Repeat the same on the other side.

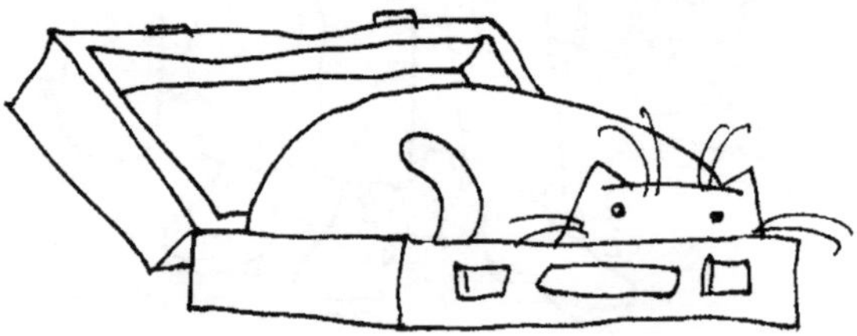

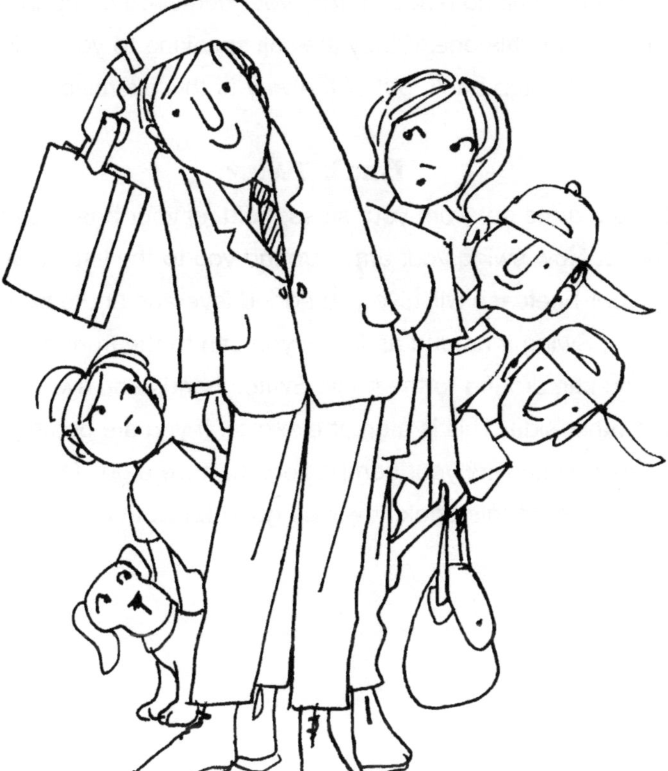

If there is still no reaction from your bemused companions you could try this one. If they are still speaking to you, ask them to step back, out of the way of this exercise.

Back Twist

Hold your arms out from your sides, holding your briefcase in your right hand. Now swing your arms around you to the left, twisting your back. Your briefcase will give you added leverage and a better back work-out. Swing it around as far as you can to the front and then as far as you can around to the back. Switch hands and swing it around on the other side. This is a great exercise. If you are getting tired at this point, invite your companions to have a go. Tell them about this book; it will be good for both of us.

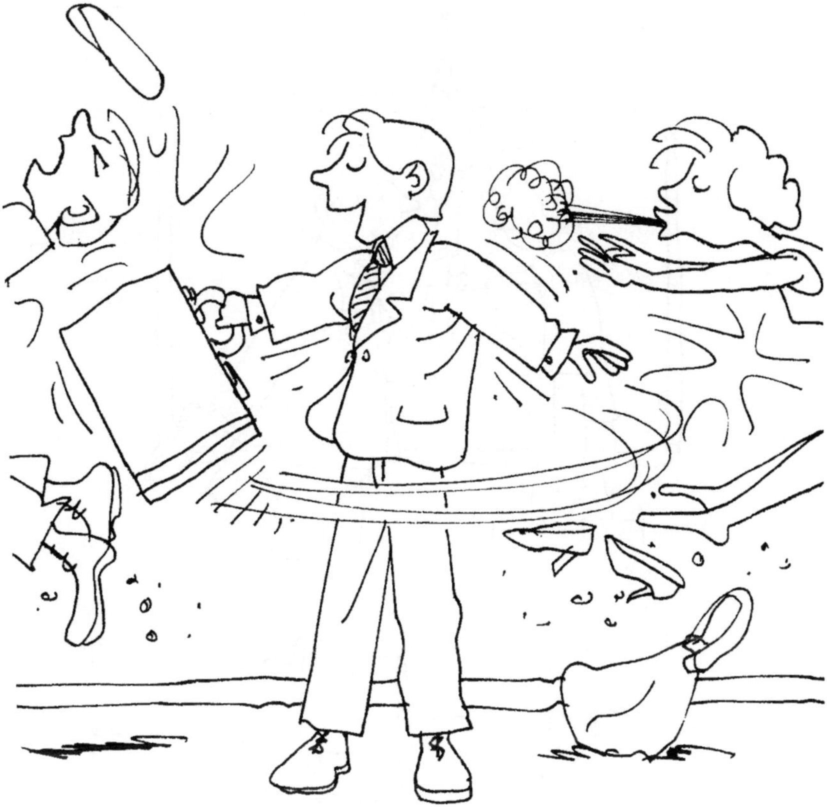

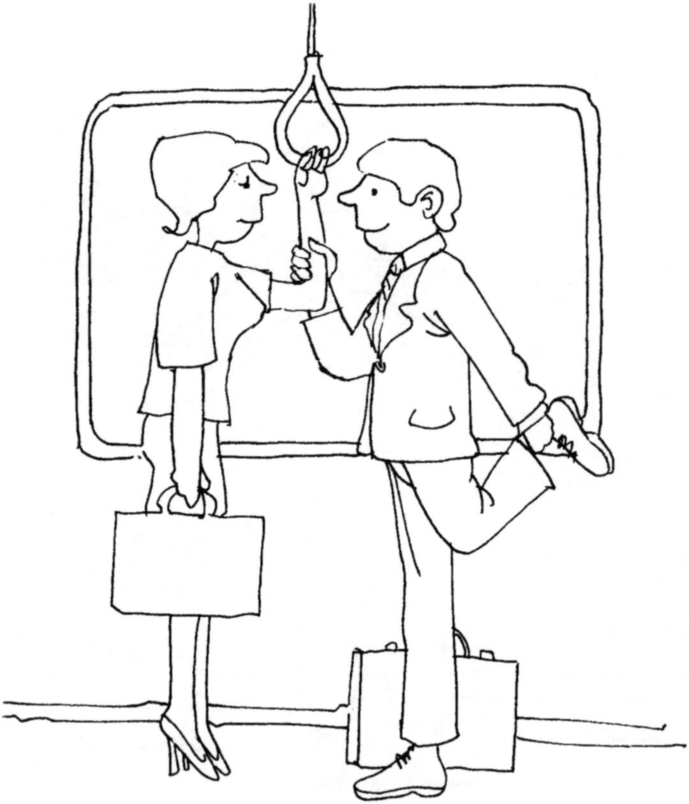

MORE STANDING STUFF

Thigh Stretch

If you are standing in a crowded train or bus, find someone or something to hold on to steady yourself. Take hold of your ankle and pull it up behind your bottom and push your thigh back in the direction your hand is pulling. This gives the thigh a really excellent stretch. Now stretch the other leg.

Don't try this in a really crowded area. People seem to get upset, complaining about their clothing getting muddy, etc. … not understanding that you exercising your thigh might be more important. Don't be put off by this attitude – explain that you're only doing it for a minute at a time. This should satisfy them.

Calf Stretch

Still holding on to what you were holding on to before, slowly bend your knees. Keep going as far as you can. Begin to feel the stretch in your calf muscles and your thighs. Think down. Try to get lower each time. Count to ten and relax back into the standing position.

Straighten your legs and back and stretch back, pulling the shoulders back and sticking out your chest. Relax, and go up on to your toes as if you are being pulled up by your hair. Count to ten to give yourself a good stretch.

Now bend your knees again. Sink lower, if you can. When you come up you may find a need to shake out your legs. If you do this, point the heel away from you to get a really full stretch.

Repeat twice to give yourself the desired *one-minute exercise*!

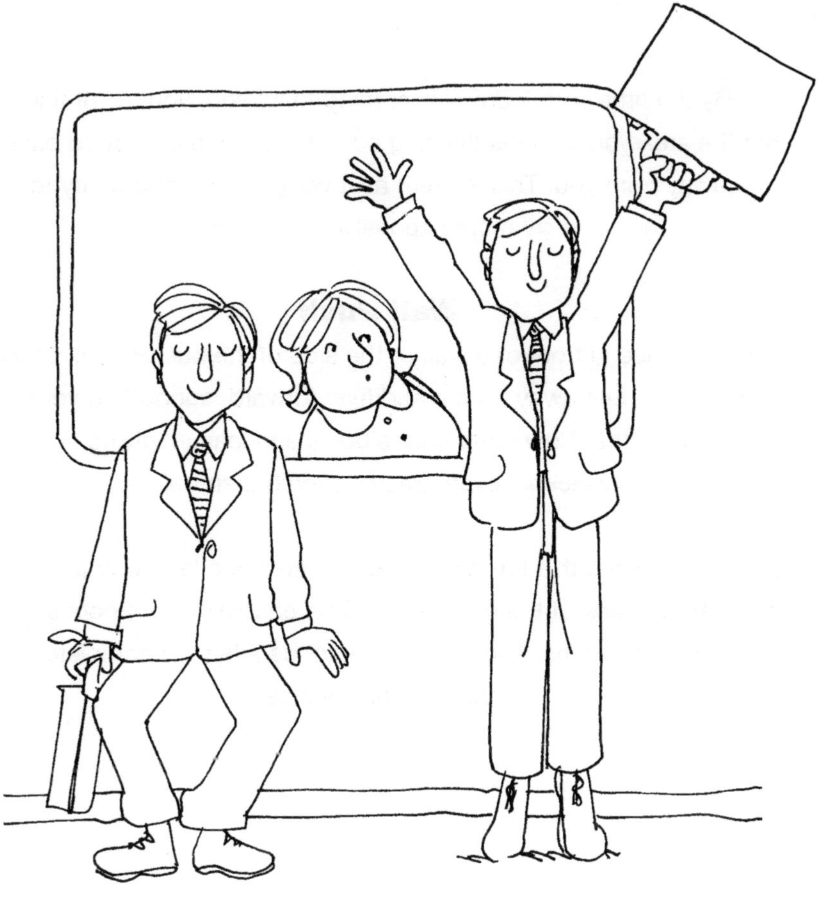

By the time your journey is coming to its end, you might find that the area you are in is thinning out. Or people may just be backing away from you. This is great as it will give an opportunity to try more expansive exercises.

Wall Push

Find a space in front of a wall or the side of the bus or train. Stand about three feet away from it and lean forward, supporting yourself with your hands. Now bend your elbows and lean in, giving your calf muscles an even greater stretch than before.

After doing this for thirty seconds, take one leg away and put it at the back of the other ankle. This enables you to concentrate on one leg at a time. These fifteen seconds a leg will complete your *one-minute exercise*!

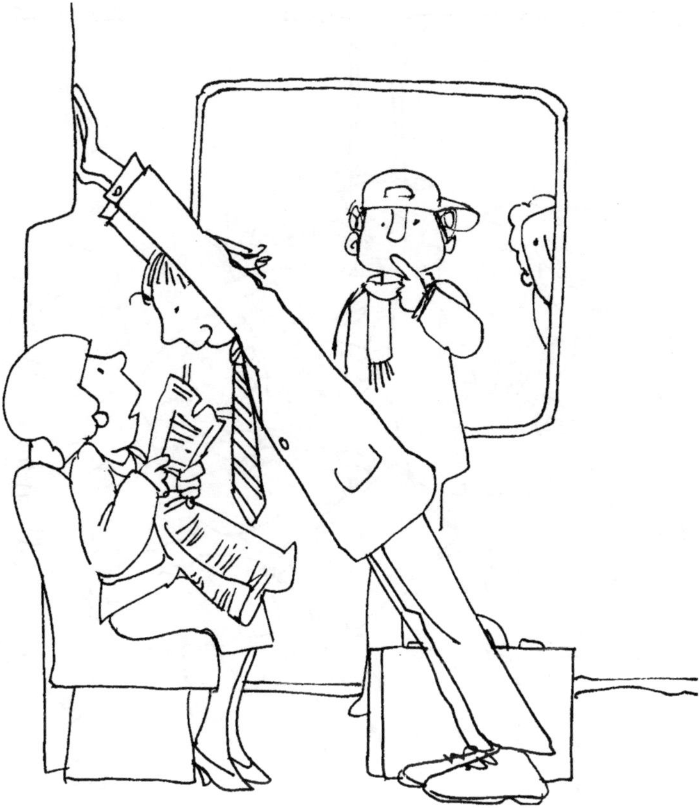

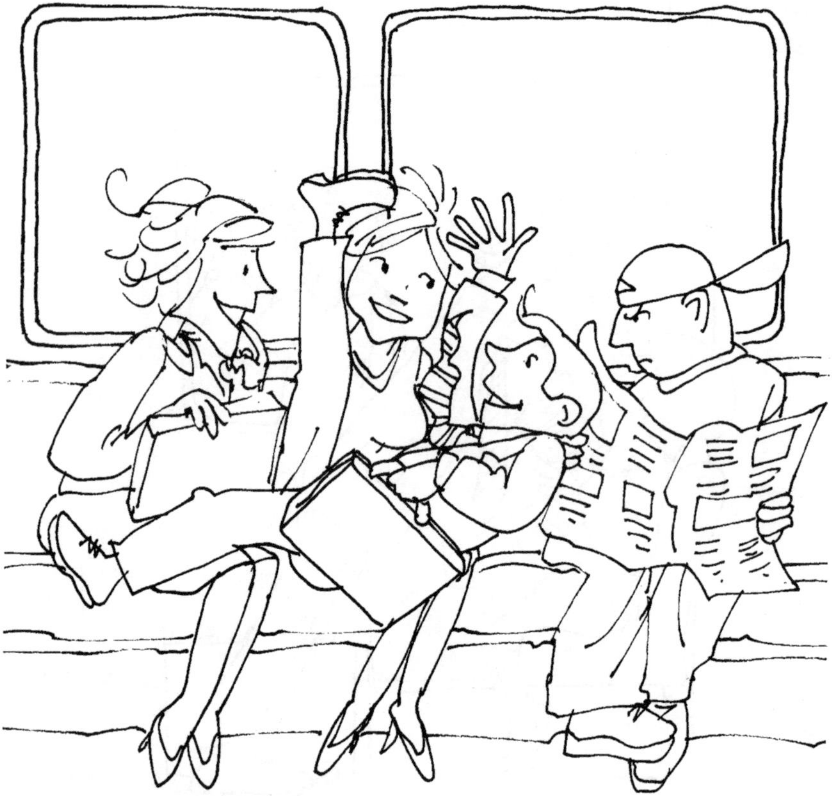

Balancing

This can be quite a challenge in a crowded bus or train, but is very good for you. Your balance gets more unstable as you get older, so the sooner you start practising it the better.

Once the bus or train gets going, try balancing on one leg. This can be quite difficult at first so hold on to something or somebody until you feel comfortable with your stance. Do equal balancing on both legs, as most people find one-leg standing is easier on one particular leg than the other. Embrace the true meaning of balance.

Once you acquire some expertise in this area, be aware of the pitfalls. Don't become over-confident. A dog, suddenly stepping into the road in front of the bus, could be the end of your exercising for ever. So be mindful of the traffic situation. Of course, it could be a way of meeting new people.

IN THE WORKPLACE

Once at work you can relax for a while. I presume that you have already run up the stairs a few times, so sit back and take it easy. Well, till the first tea break, anyway. By this time, crouching over the computer for an hour or so will have started to make your back ache. So, it's time for a stretch. Still seated, interlock your fingers and push them up above your head. Push up and back, giving the top part of your back a pop! Stand up and give your legs a shake-out. Have a cup of coffee and a chat.

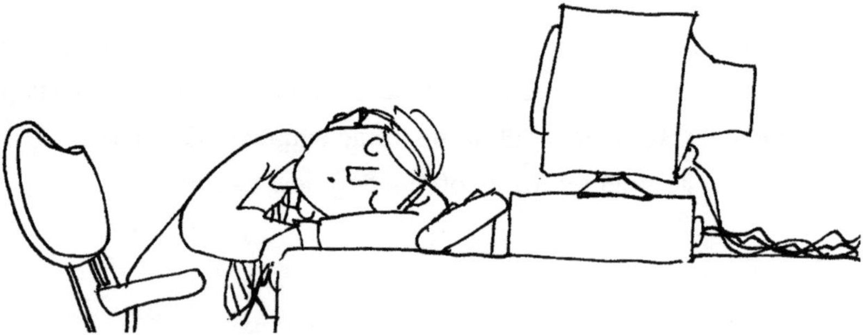

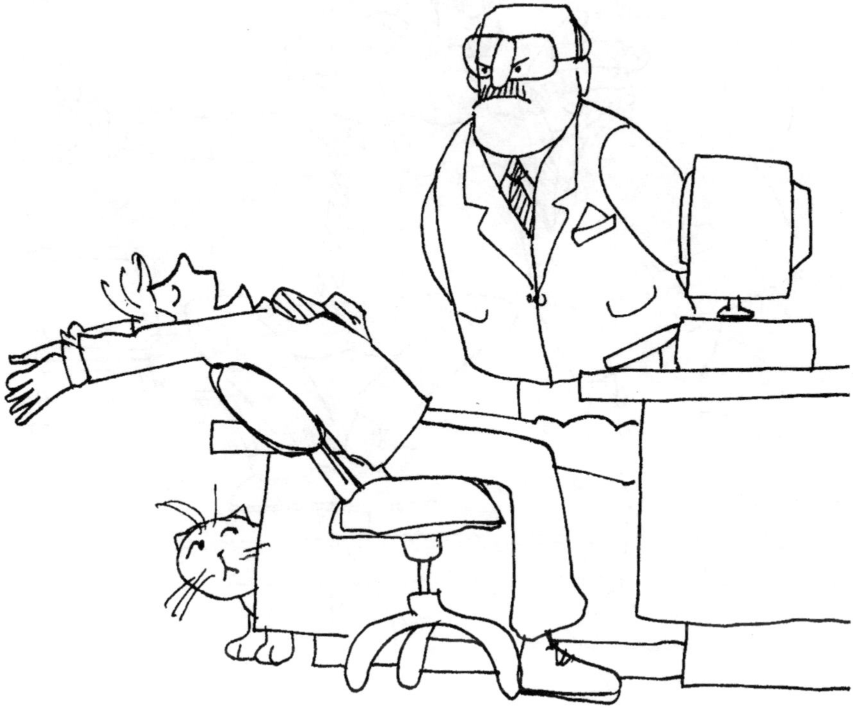

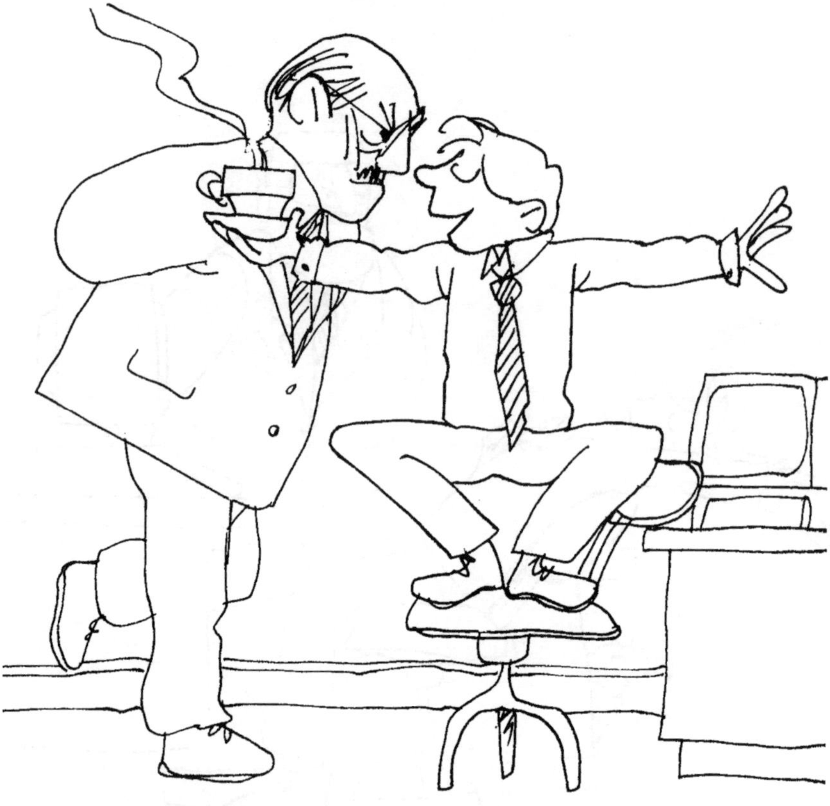

Deep Knee Bend

This is a good one to try on your coffee-break. Stand up straight. Then go into a deep knee bend. The trick is not to bend forward but to keep your back upright with your 'tail' tucked in. Holding a cup of coffee while you do this will help you keep your posture straight. To add a bit of fun to life – and we do need it – slowly sink into this position while talking to a colleague. Go down to the count of ten and up to the count of ten. Do this three times and you have your *one-minute exercise*!

Balancing Again

This would be a good time for some more balancing. Disguise your exercising by humorous antics, like balancing your cup on your head while you do knee bends and then balancing on one leg. If you get any flak from your workmates try to involve them in your exercise programme. As it's only a minute at a time this shouldn't be difficult. Show them this book and all will be revealed. You could start an inter-office one-minute exercise break every half-hour or so. The world is your ostrich.

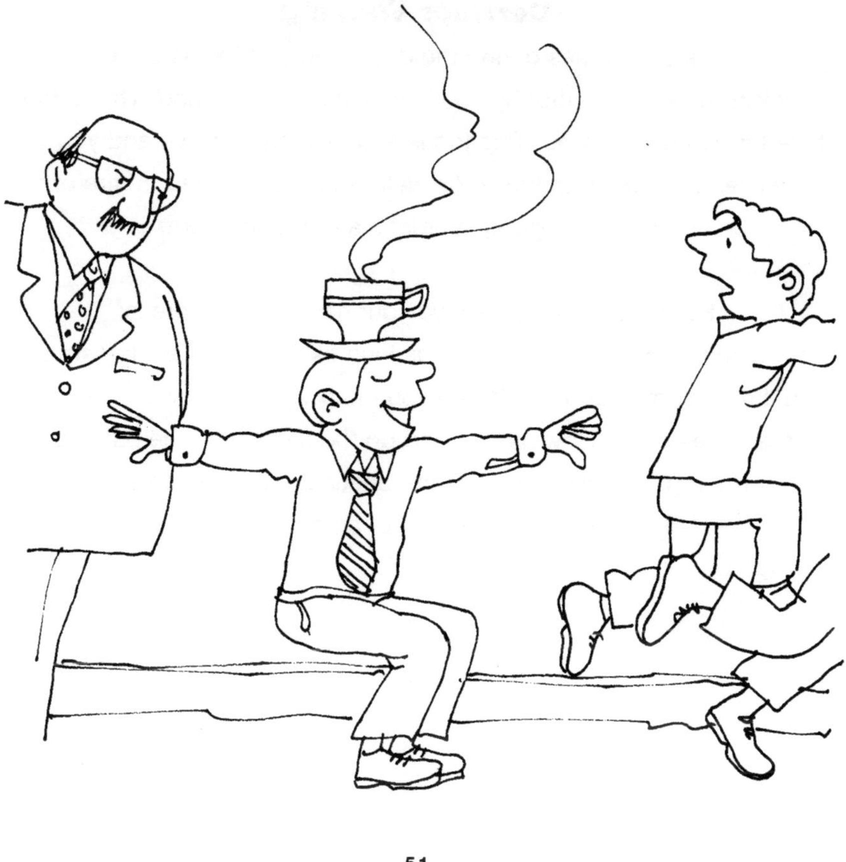

Corridor Walking

There are times during the day when you find you are walking down a corridor by yourself with no one around. This is the time for *corridor walking*. This too is a balancing exercise and you can never do enough of these. As well as improving your centre of balance, it gives your legs a good work-out.

Hold your arms up above your head at 45 degrees, for balance, and step one leg up as high as you can. Feel the stretch in the back of your thigh. When you bring your leg down, go into a deep knee bend. Now rise up and do the same with the other leg. Keep going till you reach your destination or till someone suddenly comes out of an office door.

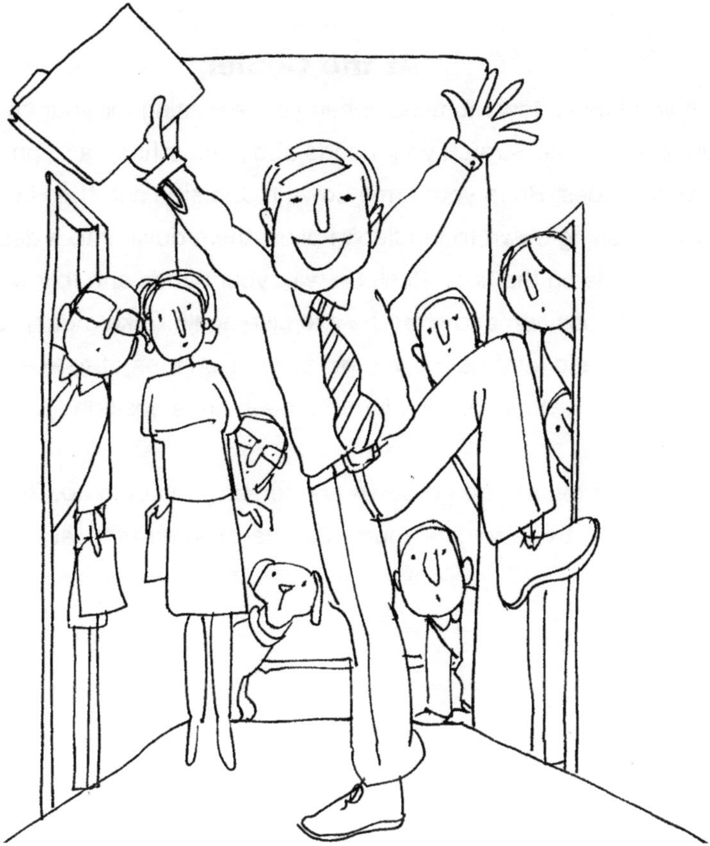

At the Copier

If you have a few moments when you're waiting for your copies to appear, try this. Stretch your hands above your head and push up on to your toes. Bring your arms down to the side and then in front of you, pushing down to the floor. Follow them down into a deep knee bend, heels on the floor. Push up with your hands and follow them up to the first position and start the exercise again. Take a deep breath as you go up and let it out as you go down. Don't forget to keep your tail in as you sink into the deep knee position.

Count ten as you go down and ten as you come up. Repeat twice to give yourself a *one-minute exercise*!

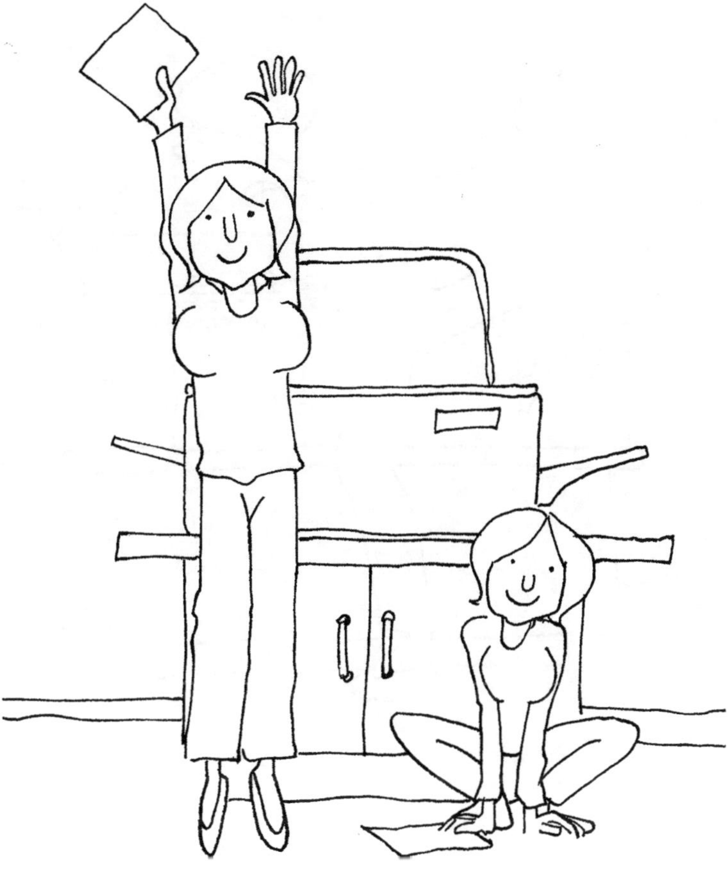

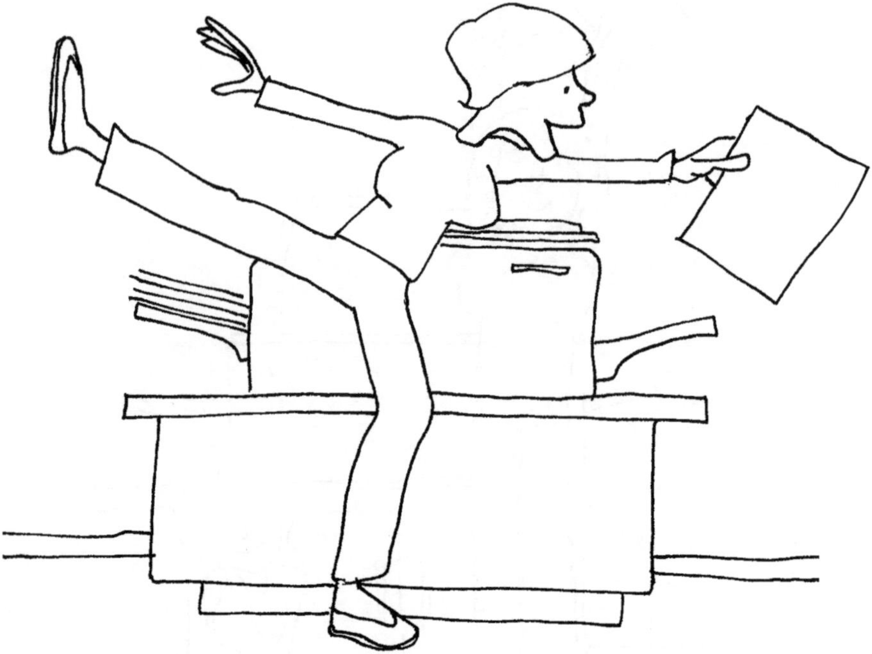

Another Copier Exercise

My old copier has to be hand-fed. So if you have a similar copier, or have to hand-feed your machine at some time, this neat exercise is excellent.

If you are feeding your copier from the left, swing your weight over to your right foot, lifting the other foot into the air. Balance here for a moment as you push the paper in. Then, as the copy paper goes through the machine, swing your weight on to your left foot and lift your right foot into the air, collecting the copy as it appears on the right. You can do this exercise any time you have to do a similar job or movement. Your timing will depend on how many copies will be required, of course, but I think it is time for a little flexibility. You can't be too rigid when other people are involved.

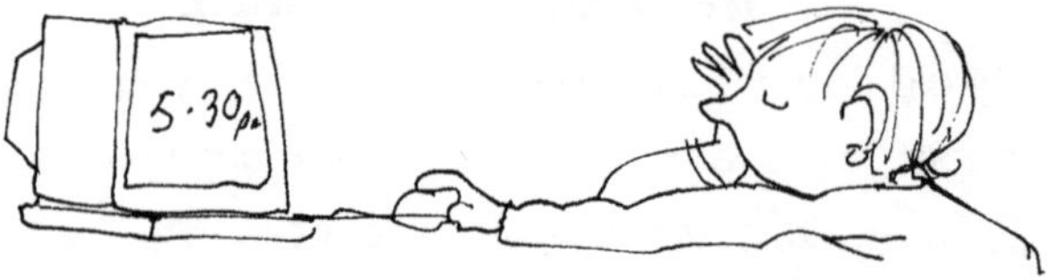

AT THE END OF THE WORKING DAY

After a full day in the workplace you will be feeling tired and, I expect, aching from being crouched over your computer all day. So go through the stretching exercises that I've mentioned in the earlier part of this book, including the How-to-Wake-up-in-the-Morning Exercise, ready for your journey home.

Sometimes I get an ache in the middle of the top of my back which is very difficult to shift, but I have found a way.

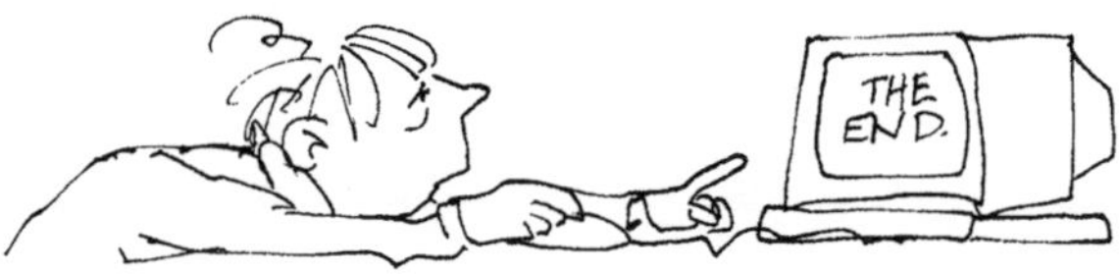

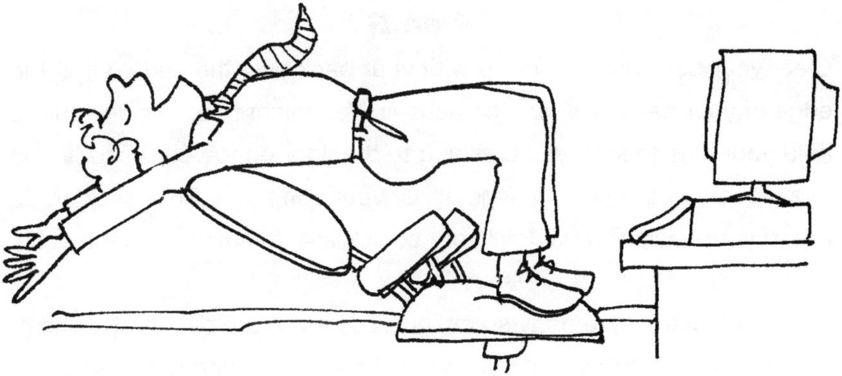

Back Clicking

Plan A

Sitting in your chair, stretch up and back, leaning into the top of the chair at the point where the ache is. You can even lift your bottom off the chair, if it will stand up to it. This will give you a little more pressure to click your backbone into where it ought to be.

If this doesn't work go to ...

Plan B

Clear your desk and lie on top with your back over the end so that the edge of your desk is where the ache is. You might need a colleague to hold your legs to stop you crashing to the floor on to your head. If you are alone try sticking your legs under your computer. Push your arms above your head and back till your back clicks free to relieve the ache.

This is an extreme remedy so only try this if you are desperate. There is also the possibility that you may be interrupted and may find your position difficult to explain.

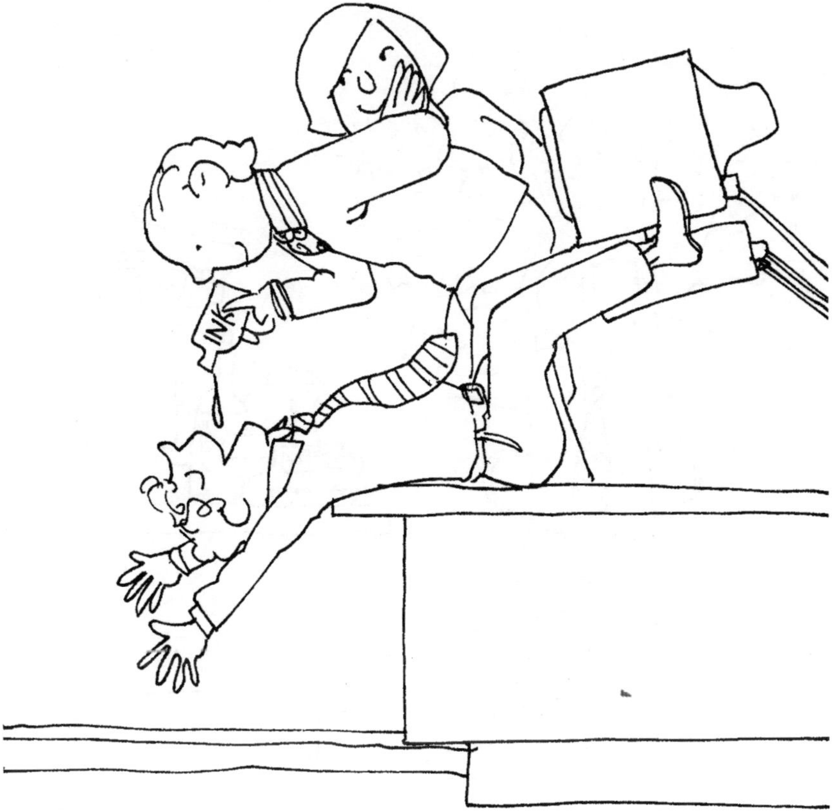
INK

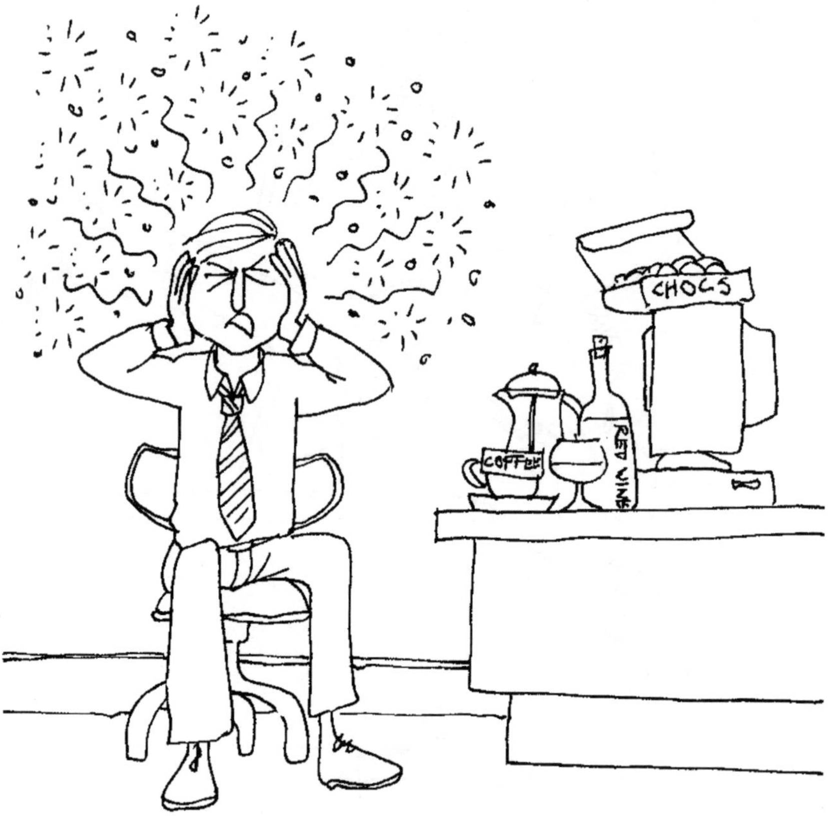
CHOCS
COFFEE
RED WINE

HEADACHES

Most headaches are the result of stress, tiredness or plain overwork – working too long without taking a break. The best way to cope with them is to avoid the conditions that seem to cause them. Easy to say, but if you know that when you work for too long at your desk you tend to get headaches, then it is better for you not to work too long at your desk and to take regular breaks.

The exercises in this book, if practised regularly, should be helpful in giving you relief from any headaches you have already.

Headaches in the forehead are often associated with constipation. Those in the back of the head are often the first signs of a cold. If you get migraine-type headaches you should check whether your intake of foods such as chocolate, coffee or red wine are the trigger for your migraines.

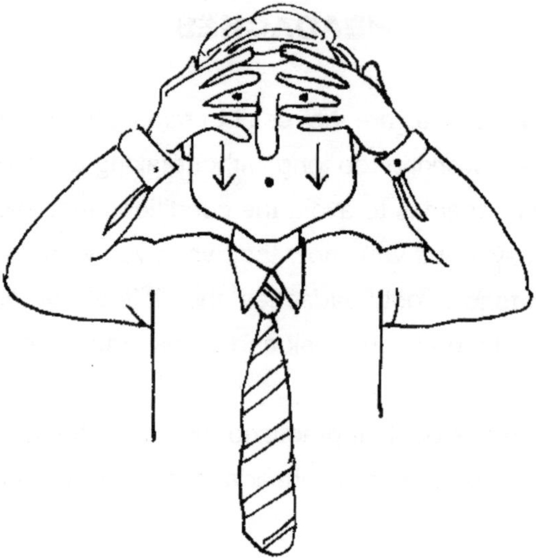

Headache Remedy

There is no magical cure for your headache but one very simple remedy is to gently massage the whole of your face with your fingers. Use smooth downward strokes to stimulate the blood circulation. Add to this massaging your neck, shoulders and back.

Get a friend or partner to help you do this.

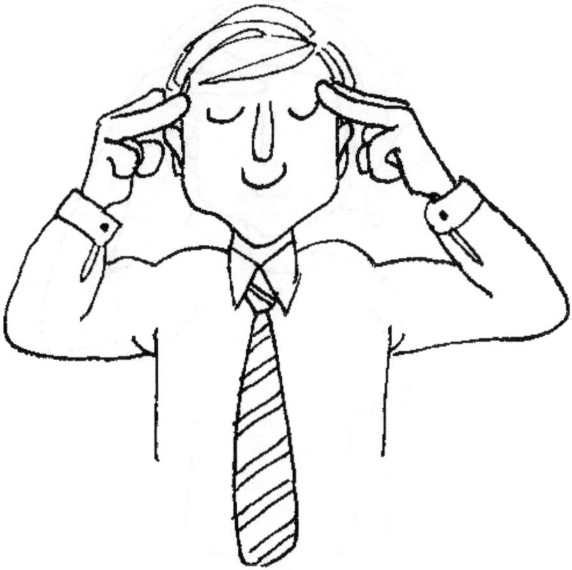

Acupressure

To relieve pain around the forehead, press firmly into the fleshy areas above the ends of your eyebrows. Using the tips of your index and middle fingers, keep the pressure on for the count of ten, then relax it. Repeat until your headache eases. Six times will ease it in a minute.

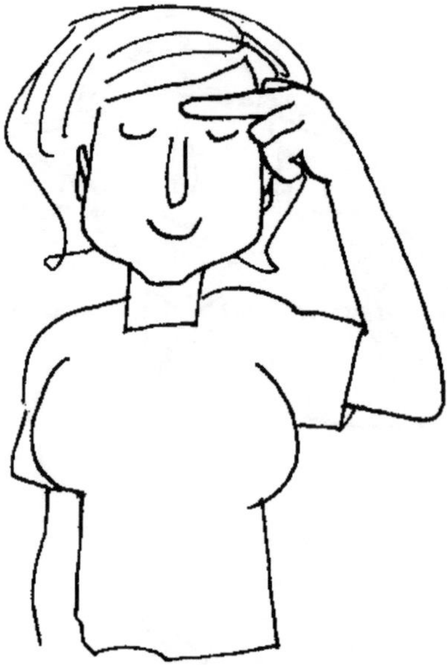

Third Eye

Place the tip of your middle finger on the spot above the ridge of your nose and below the centre of your forehead. Press firmly for the count of fifteen, then relax the pressure. Repeat three times to give yourself a *one-minute exercise* for headache relief.

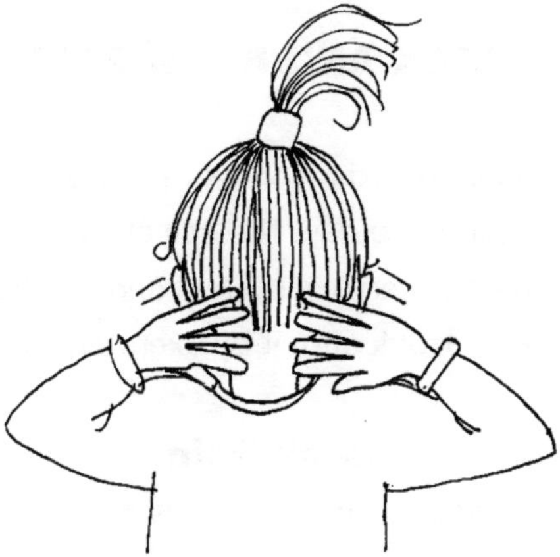

Beat the Drum

This exercise affects the twin acupoints on either side of your cervical vertebrae. Place your hands on either side of your head with your fingers flat on the back of your neck. Drum your fingers at the base of your skull for a count of sixty. This should relieve any pain you have at the back of your head.

If this doesn't feel enough, the next time pat the head to give a little more pressure. Another *one-minute exercise* for headache relief.

NECK AND BACK PAIN

The stress and fatigue of a day's work can leave you with neck and back pain for the rest of the day. The spinal column is the protective housing for the central nervous system and is often the source of aches and pains. So look after it by exercising it when you can.

Neck Pain

You can do this exercise in the train or bus, or in your car when stuck in traffic. Place your hands on your forehead, fingers flat against your head. Now push your head forward, using your neck muscles. Don't push back with your hands. It's your neck that's getting the work-out, not your hands. Count to ten and relax. Repeat five times, keeping an eye on the traffic as you do. This will give you your *one-minute exercise*. Repeat when you can during the journey home.

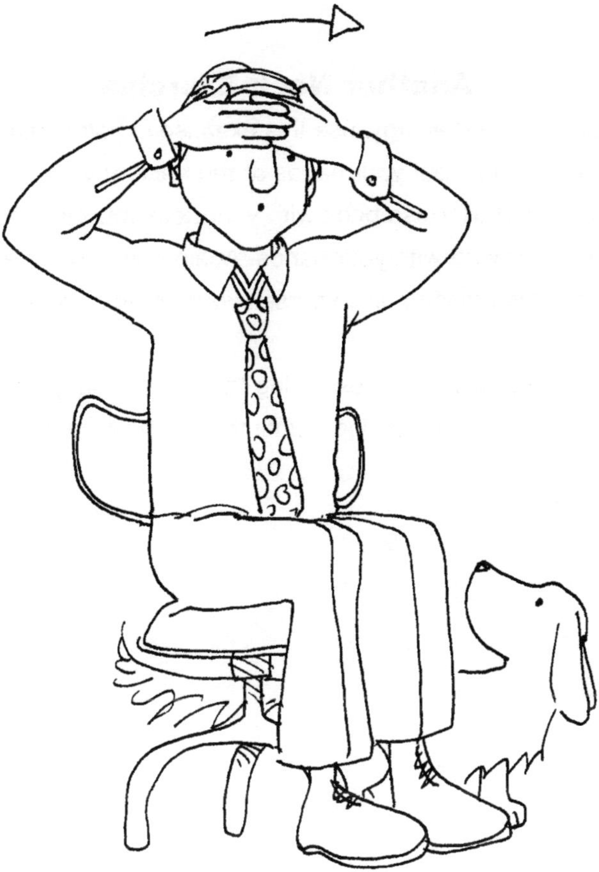

Another Neck Exercise

If you have time and energy, use this exercise in combination with the previous one. Now put your hands at the back of your head, at the base of your skull. Push back with your neck muscles. As before, don't push forward with your hands. Again count to ten and relax. Repeat five times to give yourself your *one-minute exercise*.

Combine these two exercises during the rest of your journey home, and keep repeating it until the aching recedes.

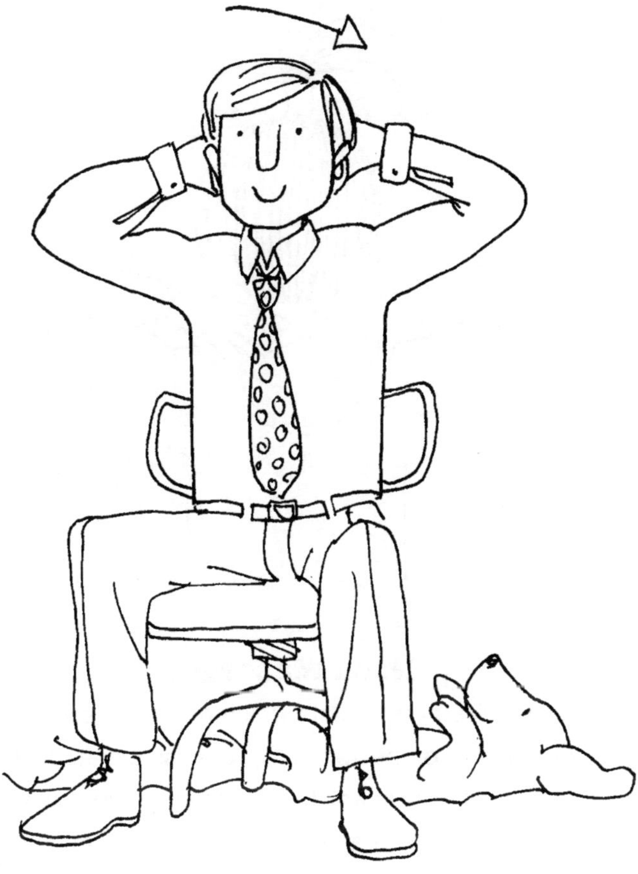

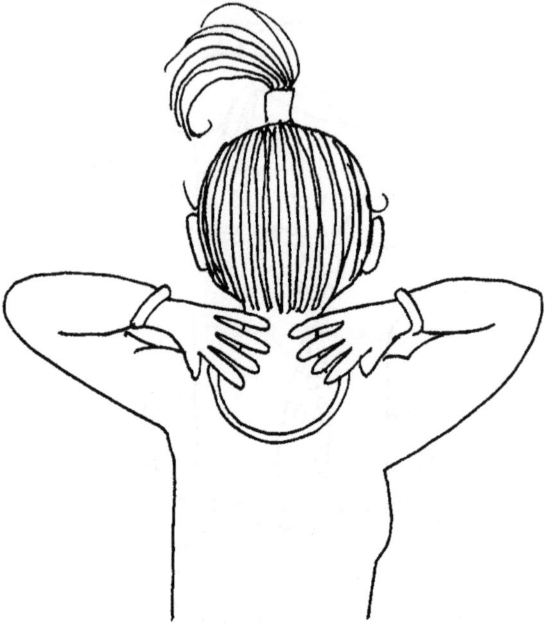

Neck Massage

There is a series of acupoints which run down each side of the neck at the top of the spine. If you massage them with your fingertips you will relieve any tension there. You should do this for a whole minute at a time to get the full benefit.

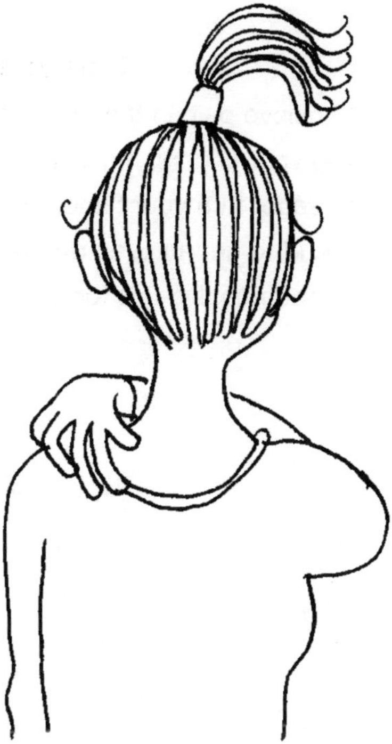

Shoulder Massages

You should feel much better after massaging your neck. Now we come to your shoulders. Using your right hand, massage the back of your left shoulder. There is usually a lot of tension in this area, so work your fingers in as hard as you can stand, digging them deep into the muscles. Now work the other side. If you are in your car, don't be tempted to do this exercise on the move. You need to concentrate on what you are doing. A full minute on each side will give you a great work-out.

Lower Back Massage

To relieve pain in the mid to lower back area, sit upright on a stool. Using your fingers, massage either side of your spine. To get a deeper massage, turn your hands over and use the knuckles of your fingers. And to get an even deeper massage, use the knuckles of your thumbs. Do this for a full minute at a time for a good result.

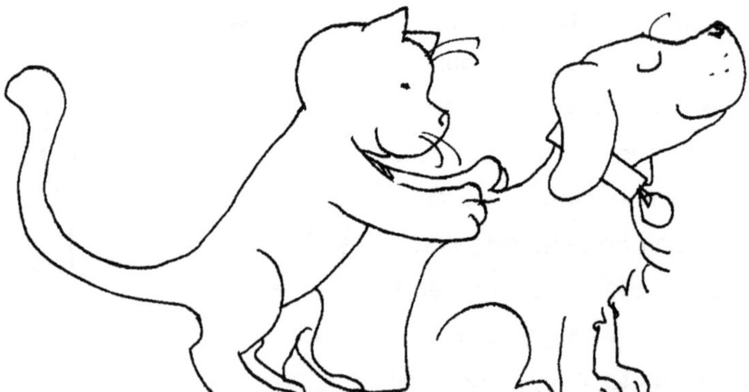

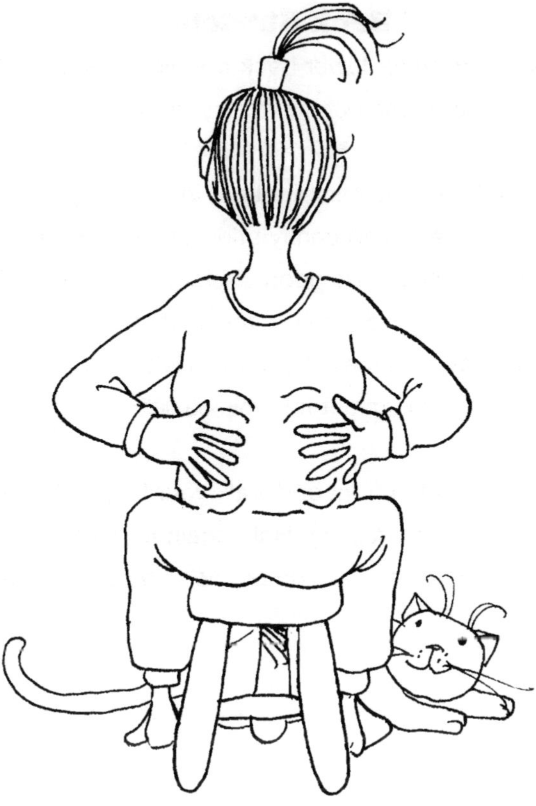

Back Stretch

This is a good exercise for lower back troubles. Better wait until you get home before you try this one.

Sit on the floor with your legs straight out in front of you. Stretch your arms up above your head and gently bring them forward to touch your toes, giving your back a really good stretch. Hold this position for a count of five. If you can't reach your toes, just bend your legs a little so you can. Repeat five times. Try it again with your legs crossed – you might find this easier.

Stretch your hands out in front and walk your fingers forward. Go as far as you can without straining. Hold again for a count of five and repeat five times, for another *one-minute exercise*.

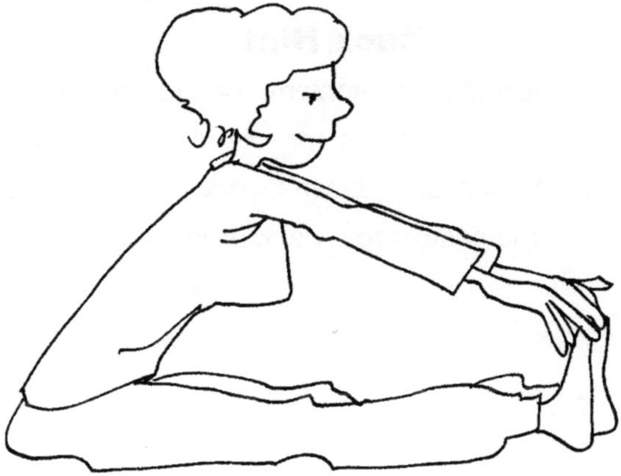

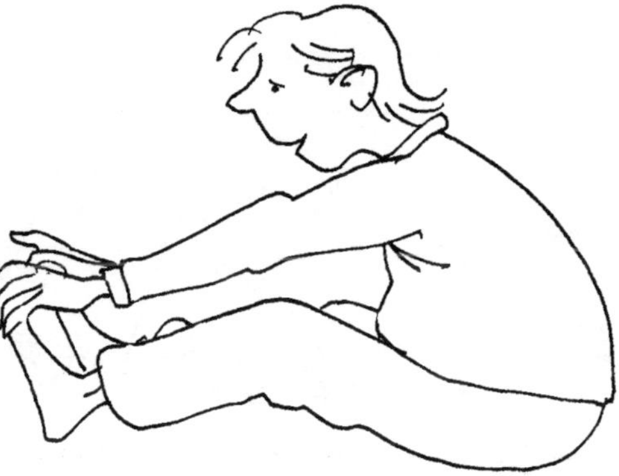

Back Hint

If you have a continual back problem, try and find a pilates class near you. They specialise in this sort of problem. Or have a word with your doctor if pilates doesn't work. Exercise is usually the answer to a back problem.

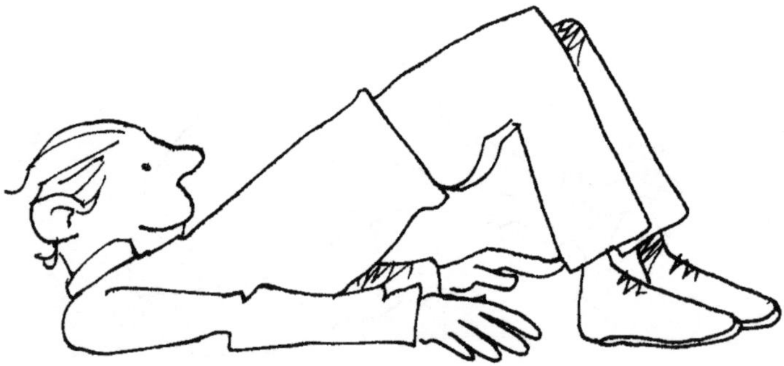

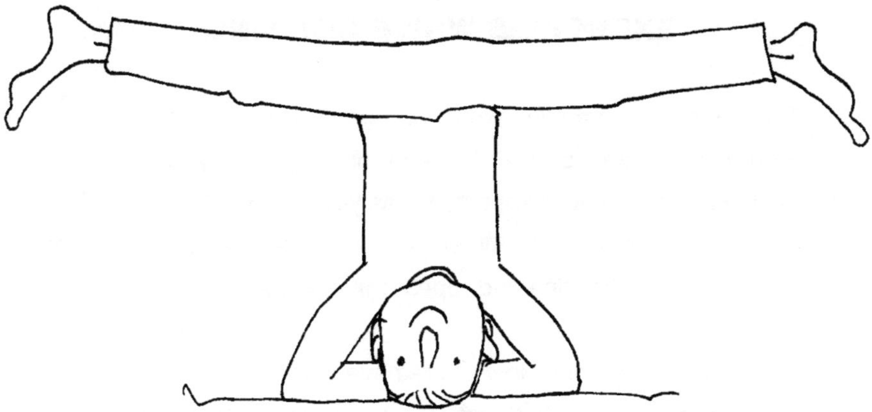

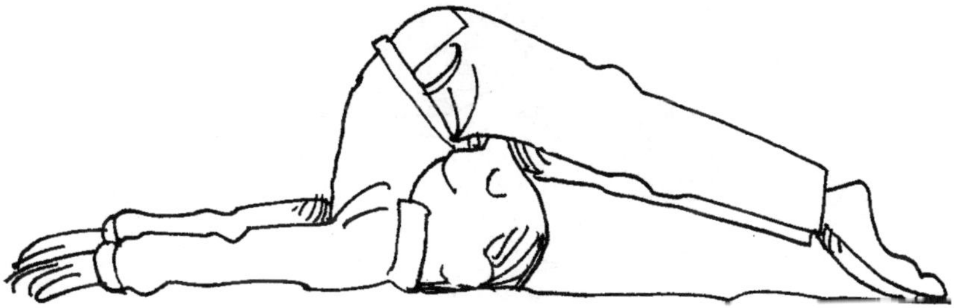

EXERCISES WHILE COOKING

There is a lot of standing when you are cooking so there is an opportunity for exercising. Balance on one leg while you chop the vegetables, bending your knee as far as you can. Feel the stretch in your calf and thigh muscles. When your leg tires, change over to the other one and repeat the exercise.

If you have to bend down to retrieve something from the floor or to pop something into the oven, don't bend forward. Do a full squat with your heels on the floor.

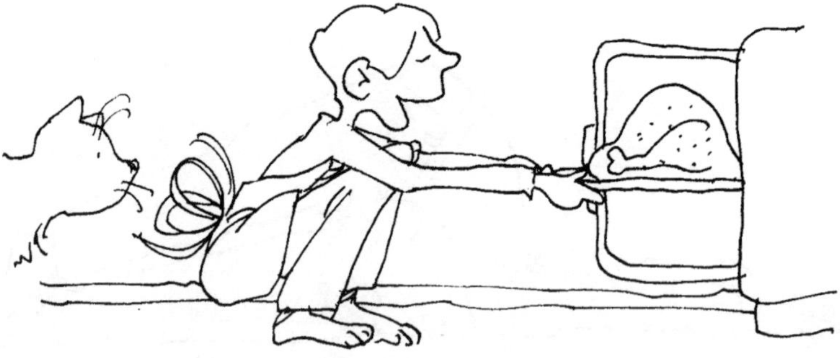

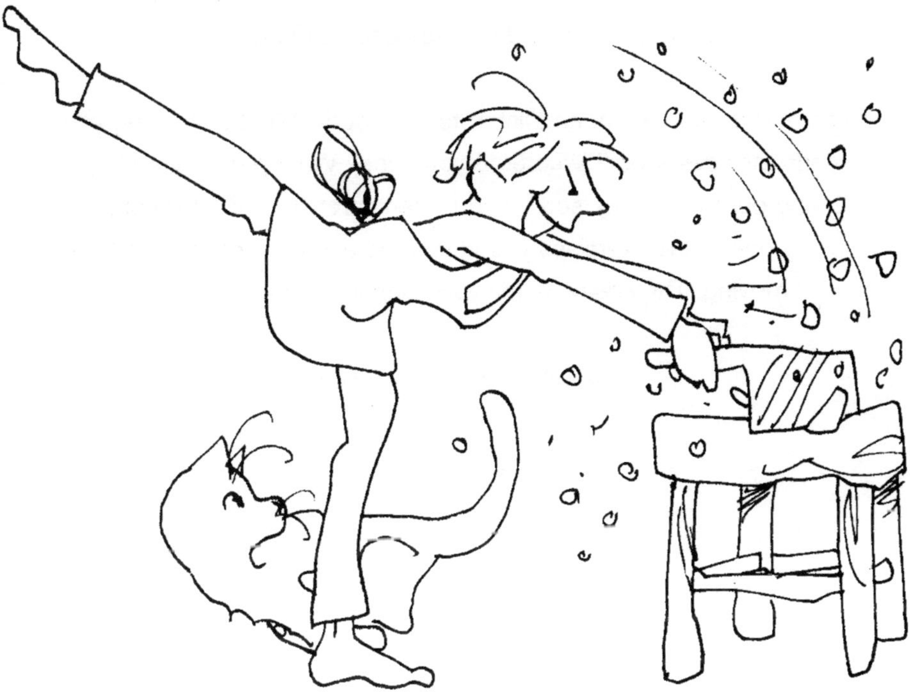

Fast Food

If you are a microwave owner, you will have lots more time for exercise. As microwaves cook whole meals in a matter of minutes, don't waste time, get going.

Just stand for a moment and listen to your body. What is it telling you it needs (besides food)? Where do you ache? What part of your body is crying out to be exercised? If you listen carefully, it will tell you. So using one of the exercises you have tried already, get your body moving. Then relax, enjoy your dinner and have a rest.

Try to get a good night's sleep.

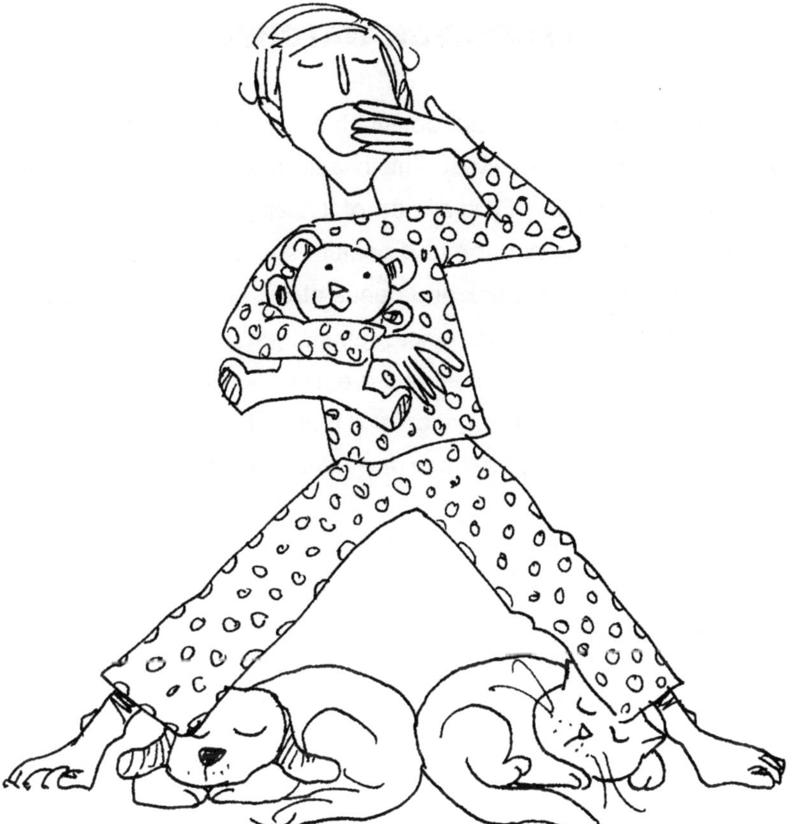

TELEVISION WATCHING

Constipation, indigestion, obesity and other related problems are now common in the West. This is a lot to do with our unsuitable lifestyle, and watching TV is all part of it. Being slumped on a couch for hours at a time is bad for your posture and your digestive system. Get up when there is a break and dance about. Jumping is good, as is running on the spot or jogging into the kitchen to make a cup of tea. Stretching and deep breathing are all good exercises to do. It's inactivity for hours on end that is the problem so get going on those *one-minute exercises*!

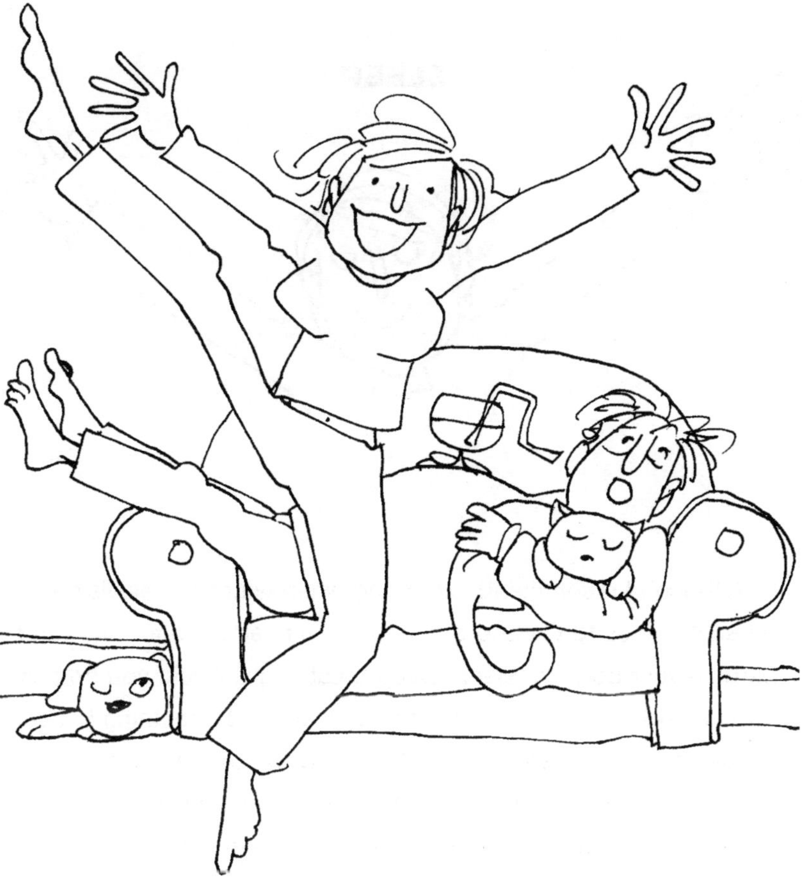

SLEEP

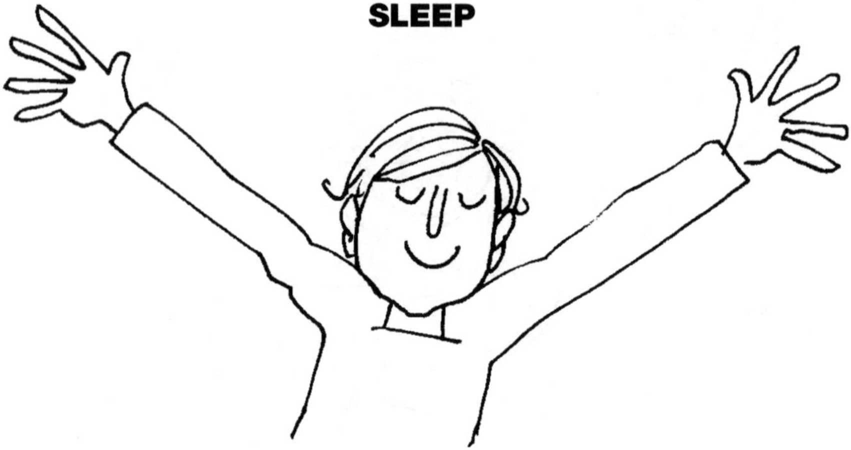

Although I recommend exercising when watching television, when it comes to the end of the day you need to wind down and prepare your body for sleep. Deep breathing will help you do this. Stand up and stretch your arms above your head, breathing in deeply as you do so. Now bring your arms down to the sides and breathe out. Remember to breathe in expanding your stomach before filling your lungs. Repeat five times.

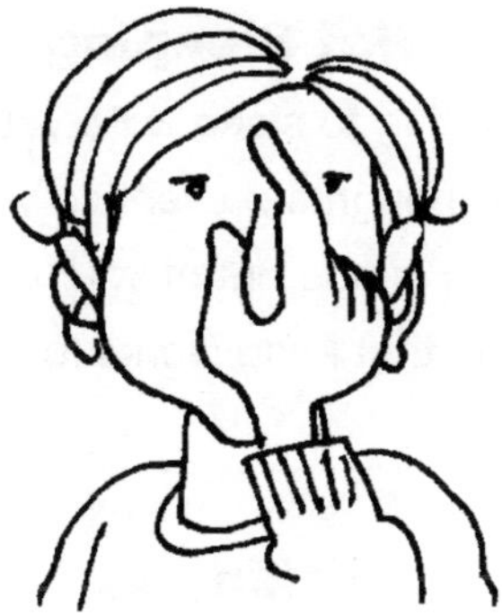

Breathing

If you are sitting down and can't get your back off the couch, try this. Rest your elbow on the back of your hand and put your index finger on your forehead between your eyes. Close your right nostril with your right thumb and inhale slowly until your stomach and lungs are full, hold for a second or two, then exhale just as slowly until the air has gone. Now release your right nostril and close your left one, using your right middle finger. Breathe in and out as before. Count to ten while inhaling and use the same count for exhaling. Repeat twice.

Not Sleeping

If you have trouble getting to sleep, with your mind going over the day's events and other thoughts preventing you from dropping off, try 'looking' at the air going in and out of your nostrils. This is a method used in meditating that I find works for a wonderful sleep.

Waking up

If you fall asleep and then wake in the middle of the night, try this exercise. You can do this lying in your bed. Place your left ankle on your right knee. Grip the outside of the foot with your right hand and press your thumb firmly into the area just under the ball of the foot towards the centre. Maintain the pressure for a count of ten, relax and repeat on the other foot. Repeat twice on each foot. If you still can't get to sleep, there is always counting sheep jumping over a farm gate. My granny swears by this one.

SEX

Sex is an excellent exercise (as I expect you know) and very commendable for a good night's sleep afterwards. But remember, not *too soon* afterwards! This could antagonise a partner and result in a great loss of 'house points' for you.

If you are getting really keen on exercising, try adding some press-ups when it's your turn on top, or stretching if you are underneath.

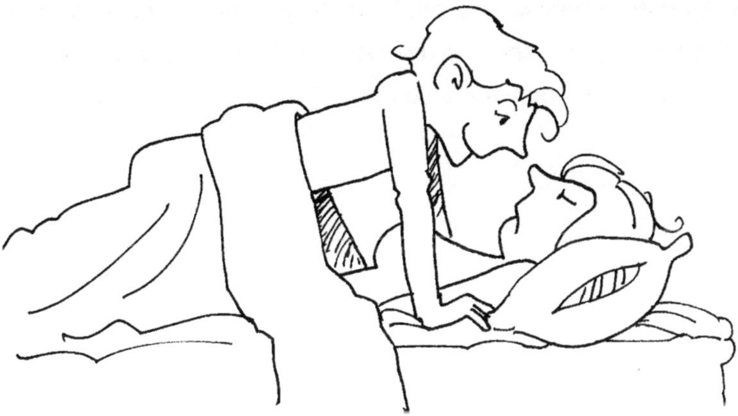

KEEPING UP THE EXERCISES ...

After your first night reading *The One-Minute Exercise Book*, getting up shouldn't be the problem it might have been the day before. You should be excited about starting your short, sharp exercises. You know they won't take long and you'll feel great after doing them so get going and *start*!

Remember how you felt yesterday after you did the How-to-Wake-up-in-the-Morning Exercise? Go on, try it. Why wouldn't you want to feel better, refreshed, enlivened, rejuvenated, reinvigorated, revitalised and like you felt when you were a young child? You can do it! *Just start!*

TO SUM UP

Although I have approached this book humorously, there is a serious intent. Obesity, indigestion, constipation and other related problems to do with our digestive system are becoming extremely common. It is inactivity and our sedentary lifestyle that is likely to be the cause of our digestive troubles, so the first step is to start taking regular exercise. So use this book to get you started.

You will start to feel better almost immediately and the more you do the better you will feel, even in a short burst of a minute at a time. Stick at it and do some exercise every day. Do some *now*, while you are reading this book.

Here's to your good health! Good luck!